THE METAPHOR TOOLBOX

SCRIPTS AND STORIES FOR HYPNOTHERAPISTS, COUNSELLORS AND COACHES

DEBBIE WALLER, EDITOR

Cover image: Vitalii Bashkatov (iStockphoto), image composite by David Waller.

Paperback ISBN: 978-1-7391573-0-2

OTHER TITLES BY DEBBIE WALLER

The Hypnotherapist's Companion: a practical guide to practice

Their Worlds, Your Words: the hypnotherapist's guide to effective scripts and sessions

The Hypnotherapy Handbook. Ed: Ann Jaloba (contributor)

All available from Amazon in paperback and on kindle

Or you can buy direct from the author via www.debbiewallerauthor.co.uk

DISCLAIMER

The information in this book is not intended as a substitute for medical/psychological advice, nor for appropriate training and supervision in the therapeutic use of metaphors.

The content, information, opinions, advice, and metaphors included in this book are based on the authors' own experiences. We do not know you or your clients, so cannot vouch for their efficacy or suitability in any specific situation. if you wish to use them for yourself, or with others, you take full responsibility for your actions.

All content is for information only and is not warranted for accuracy or any other implied or explicit purpose. The authors and publisher shall in no event be held liable for any direct, indirect, incidental, or other damages of any kind arising directly or indirectly from the use of the information contained in this book.

Every effort has been made to trace or contact all copyright holders. The publishers will be pleased to make good any omissions or rectify any mistakes brought to their attention at the earliest opportunity.

CONTENTS

CHAPTER THREE
Finding inner strength and resilience

CHAPTER FOUR
Clearing Metaphors

CHAPTER FIVE
Fairy tales and the wisdom of old wives

INTRODUCTION
AMAZED APPRECIATION

This book was conceived as a celebration of the tenth anniversary of my training school, Yorkshire Hypnotherapy Training. I could have decided to write the whole thing myself, of course, but I felt that it was better to showcase the work of those who have been involved with the school over those years, so here it is... our anthology of metaphors.

Some of the authors have been trained by YHT, and others have completed CPD courses or supervision with us, but all are generous, creative, and wonderful people who contributed their voices to help mark our birthday.

I am constantly amazed by the talents of those who pass through our doors and have no doubt you will be hearing more about all of those featured here, as they continue and grow within their careers. Some have already authored books of their own, and no doubt others will do so in the future. Many support other therapists as well as seeing clients, so watch out for them as speakers, supervisors, and authors.

To those who have begun or continued their careers with Yorkshire Hypnotherapy Training. It's wonderful to see your careers develop and thank you for all you taught me along the way.
'When one teaches, two learn.' Robert Heinlein

FOREWORD

MARION ROBB

Once upon a time, in a chilly land, with many stony mountains capped with snow, a child was born, and thus began the story of her life – a life encircled and interwoven with thousands of stories. There were beautiful stories, heart-breaking stories, family tales, cultural or religious morality plays and, sometimes, prettily embroidered tales of her own life events.

These stories did not just form a linear record which would ultimately provide a history for the adult-to-be, but over time formed a never quite completed tapestry of many threads, full of beautiful colours, tragic scenes, magical events, complex stitches, and every emotion known to humankind. So beautiful was this tapestry with all its panels forming stories and patterns, and all its hidden connections behind the cloth which led from one tale to the other, that it really was a work of art.

Sometimes, some of these panels and pictures were eventually overlaid with a slightly different tale – a different emphasis or colour or texture – all bringing a new dimension to the tapestry. Eventually, the work became so large that images and tales had to be condensed and made easier and faster to find. It so happened that this child's tapestry had a fearsome wolf, right at its centre, denoting everything she found frightening and evil to her young mind.

The little child loved the comfort of story time, and at first, that was the simple reason she settled sleepily down to listen as her parents read book after book of fairy stories and fables. Through time, she learned to fear wolves, because of three little pigs, who were eaten, and because Little Red Riding Hood strayed from the path. However, it was some time before she understood that a wolf might not be a wolf with four legs and yellow fangs at all, but might be a competitive schoolfriend, or a boss, or that seemingly nice chap she met in the bar.

Eventually, she understood that within many of these stories were gaps, things which were not said, but implied, hidden, or even disguised. At school, in the playground, she sang a song about a Ring o' Roses as she and her friends skipped with ropes, never knowing the story was a metaphor – hiding the truth that the children falling down did so because of a dread plague, not because of a game. When the teacher told her about the stories behind nursery rhymes like Jack and Jill and Ring o' Roses, she became instantly hooked on the possibilities of metaphor.

She found her life was surrounded by stories with hidden meanings and lessons; in song, in poetry, in prose, film, conversations at the kitchen table, Sunday school, comics and newspapers, and every medium where people communicated with others. As life progressed, she became a bit of a detective, always looking underneath to see what the story truly meant and what lesson she was meant to take from it.

This, I suspect, is the story of everyone. From our first breaths, we learn about the world of people, emotion, and events from the narratives we are told, those we choose to tell, and how we choose to tell them. Even people who dislike fiction of any sort, and who would robustly deny the concept of possessing an imagination, are nevertheless exposed daily to the narratives of others. Through those everyday tales, one can understand both consciously and subconsciously that meaning may be disguised, presented, and soothed through individual metaphorical constructs.

It is certainly the story of most of the excellent hypnotherapists I have met. These therapists are fascinated by the theatre that lives in other people's minds, and the internal tapestries they develop to bind and form their own stories. They share a common understanding of how to use the metaphors and narratives the client presents, or to offer new alternatives to help them change or heal inner stories and beliefs which no longer serve them.

I am a believer in these concepts:

"The greatest thing by far is to be a master of metaphor. It is the one thing that cannot be learned from others, and it is also a sign of genius."
Aristotle

"Metaphors are not simply a linguistic or literary device; they play an important role in learning and cognitively organizing an understanding of the world (Lakoff & Johnson, 1980; Aragno, 2009; Evans, 2010)"

The metaphors a client presents are often the subconscious amalgamations and shortcuts which their minds have chosen to rationalise events, feelings, traumas, beliefs, and issues they now choose to change.

These metaphors may have been present in the client's psyche since childhood with little adaptation. They may have developed as shortcuts for the client to access feelings and memories quickly. Learning to speak to clients who are reflecting and building upon their own metaphors, can not only rapidly increase rapport and understanding of their personal worldviews and beliefs, but may also raise your work from the realms of good basic skills to something which approaches an artform in its ability to facilitate change for your clients.

I was shocked a few months ago to realise that one of my own favourite books of therapeutic metaphors, 'Stories for the Third Ear' by Lee Wallas, was first published in 1985 – long before many hypnotherapists working today were so much as a metaphorical twinkle in their fathers' eyes. Therefore, I was particularly pleased to learn that Debbie Waller was editing a volume of contemporary and modern therapeutic metaphors that have been developed and used in the practices of some of her own YHT graduates.

The book itself is both a delight and a resource, exemplifying not only the excellence in the teaching provided to these graduates, who are all now working hypnotherapists, but demonstrating diversity, intelligence, and creativity in the use of therapeutic metaphor, and providing inspiration and insight for students and seasoned practitioners alike.

Marion Robb

Marion is a well-respected member of her professional community, is well-known internationally for her role as co-moderator of the forum "Hypnotic Women" and has been a Board Member of the Scottish Hypnotherapy Foundation on several occasions. She is committed to Continuing Professional Development and has been fortunate to train with many of the world's leading hypnotists and hypnotherapists.

Marion qualified as a hypnotherapist in 2009, and as a supervisor in 2015. She has clients and supervisees worldwide. She operates out of Central Scotland, with her main premises being in Dunfermline.

CHAPTER ONE

TELLING STORIES – WHY THEY MATTER AND HOW THEY HEAL

STORIES, MEANING AND METAPHOR

AUTHOR: DEBBIE WALLER

A tale, however slight, illuminates truth.

Jalaluddin Rumi, 14th-century Persian poet, mystic and storyteller[1]

A metaphor is a form of language which describes something in terms which aren't factually accurate, to bring about an accurate sense of the thing being described. For example, saying that someone has a 'heart of stone'; literally this would be impossible, but we understand from it that they are unfeeling or without empathy.

In literary terms, metaphors are generally just a few words or sentences, and a longer tale which makes a more developed point about society or human nature is an allegory. But let's not get too bogged down in technicalities. There's a long tradition of therapists using the term 'metaphors' to cover all types of healing stories, so we're going to stick to it here.

If Rumi is right in the quote above, though, all stories might contain meanings other than the obvious, whether that was the storyteller's intention or not. It's important to know if this is true before using metaphors and stories with our clients because, if it is, it opens up all kinds of ideas that we might not have considered before.

Storytelling has been around for a long time. Since before we had writing and the internet, stories have been passed down the generations for something like 30,000 years, as forms of social bonding and affirmation, entertainment, and education. Communities of all kinds have a fund of traditional tales, myths, and fables; religious figures like Jesus, Mohammed, and Buddha and teachers like Aesop all use parables and stories to make a point. So do modern politicians and advertisers. And, of course, there are autobiographical stories; the ones we share with our friends, and the ones your clients tell you about their reasons for seeking therapy.

If a story was only a good way to keep us entertained for a while, they would probably stay almost the same with each telling. But even what we think of as traditional tales change dramatically as they travel over time and distance. That's because the context in which they are told and heard changes, and we read different things into them.

To see this in action, let's look at recent concerns around a traditional heroine, Sleeping Beauty. A beautiful princess, under a curse, falls asleep until she is woken by a kiss from a conveniently placed prince. All very sweet and innocent. What you may not know is that this is a sanitised rendering of the tale. In the original 17th century version, she is raped and impregnated with twins by a passing king whilst in her magical trance, and it's one of the babies who wakes her up by sucking a magical splinter out of her finger. But (in the story at least) that's all okay because, after some blood-thirsty shenanigans from the King's first wife that would put most modern bunny boilers to shame, by the end the princess is happily married to the father of her children.[2] The end maybe justifying the means.

I really can't see Disney making that version, can you? But, for some people, even a chaste kiss to an unconscious woman feels inappropriate rather than romantic. In 2017, a school in Newcastle was asked by one of the Mums to remove *Sleeping Beauty* from the younger children's classrooms because it showed 'inappropriate sexual role models'.[3] And a year or two later, actress Kristen Bell publicly expressed similar concerns about depictions of Snow White,[4] although the wake-up kiss in that one was a relatively recent addition. Other versions offer different ways of getting to the inevitable happy ending – which is pretty much always a heterosexual wedding to someone attractive, powerful, and royal or (preferably) all three.

Whether you agree with the objections or think they are 'political correctness gone mad', you must admit that the people raising these objections are genuinely seeing something in the subtext that they don't feel comfortable with. And if you don't get it, think about how you'd feel if the story was on Facebook and the girl was asleep or drunk instead of in a magical dream state.

I'm not trying to put you off reading fairy stories to your children here, or to say that the objectors are necessarily right. My favourite was always *Beauty and the Beast*, which could be argued to include kidnapping, Stockholm Syndrome (or Lima Syndrome, depending on which version you read), persecution of the outsider, and more. I'm just asking you to think there may be more to them than meets the eye.

Of course, there are other completely different views. To borrow from *Jurassic Park*, 'sexism in survival situations'[5] is arguably different. The princess can hardly be expected to have prepared a big sign that says, 'Please kiss me', and she might prefer an unsanctioned peck on the lips to remaining indefinitely in a kind of cryogenic suspension. Waking up to find you have twins might be more of an issue, though.

It's also argued that children can distinguish between what happens in a story and real life. They don't expect bears to live in a cottage and eat porridge, for example, or to come to London from Peru when their aunt goes into a retirement home. But the concerns that people raise are genuine and they are based on the hidden assumptions and meanings of these tales rather than on the surface chatter.

Anyhow, before I go any further down the rabbit hole of fairy story history and analysis, let's call a halt, as I hope I've made the point. Whether you remember literary criticism at school with fondness or despair, there is little doubt that context does inform storytelling. People unconsciously read themes and ideas into stories which are left unsaid by the storyteller, which is exactly why therapeutic stories and metaphors work.

Stories illustrate who we are, deliberately or otherwise, so they can be read as metaphors even if that wasn't the author's intention. Orwell, for example, intended to represent the Russian Revolution in *Animal Farm*,[6] but Tolkien always denied that *Lord of the Rings* was an allegory of the Second World War,[7] even though many have read it that way.

When the metaphorical meanings don't fit anymore, we simply change the stories so that they do. Perhaps that's why there are so many 're-imaginings' of fairy tales around. They add modern sensibilities to the tales and more self-sufficiency and independence to the protagonists, especially the female ones.

That's an important point to bear in mind when you use the metaphors and stories in this book with your clients. They're not Shakespeare or otherwise sacrosanct (sorry, authors). Read them and use them – the whole project would be pointless if you didn't. But adjust them to fit your therapeutic approach, your storytelling style and your clients' situations so they illustrate the specific changes that they're trying to make.

They should be a springboard for your ideas, not a straitjacket.

STORIES AND THE BRAIN
AUTHOR: DEBBIE WALLER

Storytelling is the most powerful way to put ideas into the world.
Robert McKee, professor[1]

Why are stories so popular as tools for teaching? In part, it's because they are more engaging and easier to remember than a list of facts or rules. When they are used as therapeutic metaphors, with a deliberate underlying healing message, they are arguably less likely to 'press the rebel button' since you are just putting an idea out there for your client to respond to rather than issuing instructions. Stories help us pay attention, understand, and focus on the information we're being given, and they give us the freedom to make our own interpretation of what's being said.

But beyond that, when we listen to a story there is more going on inside our brains than responding to auditory information.

We respond emotionally to stories, and this creates observable physical changes in the body, in terms of facial expressions, breathing rate changes and so on – think of your own response when listening to a scary, sad or happy story. (Or watching a film. They're stories as well, just a visual version.)

Listening to a well-told story causes the release of oxytocin,[2] a brain chemical involved in positive emotions and empathy, and a reduction of the stress hormone cortisol.[3]

Furthermore, it creates a kind of synchronicity between the brain of the listener and that of the storyteller. Mirror neurons create a process called neural coupling, in which the listener's and storyteller's brain waves start to match one another's. This has an ongoing beneficial effect on empathy, communication, and understanding.

Our brains use many more areas to process stories than factual communications. For example, brain scans have shown that when we are presented with a metaphorical description such as someone having 'a rough day', or being a 'sweet' person, the areas of the brain that process the relevant physical experiences (in my examples, touch or taste) are activated, as well as those that deal with verbal communication.[4] Isn't that amazing?

We can also conclude from this that the responses our clients have to the metaphors and stories we tell them are not simply something going on in their imaginations. Their emotional reactions to this internal 'virtual reality' are just as real as the ones that result from physical or social experiences and thus can help to change their attitudes, beliefs, and behaviours.

USING THERAPEUTIC STORIES AND METAPHORS

AUTHOR: DEBBIE WALLER

Beware the stories you read or tell: subtly, at night, beneath the waters of consciousness, they are altering your world.

Ben Okri[1]

M any therapists use a non-directive approach to therapy. That is, we don't tell clients how they should live their lives, or even how to meet the goals they present to us. Instead, we provide a safe and non-judgemental space for them to find their own answers.

Metaphors and stories are an ideal way to do this. They allow us to rehearse ideas and change without having to experience them in real life – a bit like a roller coaster or a horror film allows us to experience fear whilst knowing we are safe.

Clients rarely turn up at our offices with a single, clear-cut problem that is isolated from the rest of their lives. Most often there is a complex web of experiences, beliefs, feelings, thoughts, and behaviours involved, which the client is struggling to understand or cope with. Raymond Berger[2] suggests that a story provides a 'cognitive package'. In other words, it breaks things down into simpler patterns and themes that make organising responses and finding solutions easier.

9

Furthermore, because a story can be presented in a dissociated way ('a man walked down the road' rather than 'imagine you are walking down the road'), it can help to reframe ideas, and to avoid obstacles like resistance because the client isn't directly confronted or told what to think.[3]

As we've said, stories are easier to remember than many other forms of information, and sometimes the point can be reinforced by simply mentioning a catchphrase or punchline without any need to repeat the whole tale.

For example, when my youngest was about four or five we left her to amuse herself in the house while we cleaned out the garage. After an hour or so, she came out carrying a tray of drinks. Tea for me, coffee for my husband, and just the right amounts of milk and sugar. We were simultaneously impressed that she could be so thoughtful and horrified that she had risked injuring herself to make it. But it was handed over with the comment, 'You said this was a dirty job so I thought you would want a drink. But I know I'm not supposed to use the kettle, so I made it with cold water'.

And if you have never drunk tea or coffee made with cold water, I really don't recommend it.

There were, of course, other options. Cold drinks would have been one (meaning drinks that were supposed to be cold) or asking my eldest (who was seven years her senior and allowed to use the kettle) to help. But the solution she'd found seemed to do the trick, so she used it.

I use this now and then to illustrate to clients how the unconscious, like a child, tends to go for the first solution it sees to a problem, rather than the best one. If anxiety does the job of keeping you safe, you'll get anxiety, even if there are other ways of doing the same job that are better and more convenient to live with. Therapy is there to help you find those better ways.

And, after the first telling, if I want to encourage the client to think past their first, knee-jerk response, I can ask something like, 'Are you making tea with cold water here?' and they know exactly what I mean. The humour can also be useful for getting past that frustrating feeling of being stuck.

Furthermore, the same story will elicit different thoughts from different people. Are you familiar with the 'Control Room' metaphor? Essentially, you ask you client to enter an imaginary room which contains all kinds of controls, find the one that is relevant to why they have come for therapy, and adjust it. So, you may turn confidence up, or anxiety down. I'm sure you can see how this works, and recommend you try it if you haven't already.

If you do this, the control rooms that they come up with are all very individual. Some aren't even rooms. The controls vary in the way they look and work, how hard they are to adjust and just about everything else. You get a similar variety in the visual representations of parts if you use that technique. They all have unconscious significance and meaning to the client in front of you.

Here's another example. How did you understand the title of this article, 'telling stories'?

- Is it literally about telling stories and, if so, in what way?
- Does it mean fibs?
- Is it an album by Tracy Chapman or an autobiography by Tim Burgess?
- Are the stories you're about to hear 'telling' in themselves – revealing, significant or persuasive?

If you took it at face value, possibly the first option was the only one you considered, and context could help you rule out references to songs and books, but the others are all valid in the right circumstances. Clients will do the same with your stories and metaphors; they will make them their own and take from them the meaning they need to heal.

BECOME A BETTER STORYTELLER

AUTHOR: DEBBIE WALLER

The purpose of a storyteller is not to tell you how to think, but to give you questions to think upon.

Brandon Sanderson, fantasy and science fiction writer [1]

You might have noticed that all the references to the physical, social, and emotional benefits of using stories and metaphors talk about 'a well-told story', so I'm going to finish here with a few pointers for those who want to improve their storytelling skills.

We're mostly focussing here on how to tell other people's stories, of course, whether you are reading them or relaying them from memory. We'll get to creating your own in just a minute.

Personalisation and scene setting

Remember that the same story will elicit different responses from different people, but they need to identify with it for that to happen. You can do this by adding words or phrases that your client used, or basing a story around their hobby, but also with a simple introduction like:

'What you said about your situation made me think of something I read in the paper the other day ...'

Or I might say it's a book I read to my kids if it has a fairy tale format, or whatever else sets the scene. The client instantly thinks 'This is about me'. In around twenty years of using this framework, I have only ever had one person say to me 'You didn't just read that in the paper, did you?' – and it worked anyway.

Prioritise emotions

Keep your focus on the emotions and the journey the client wants to make, not the literal situation. Just because the client wants to quit smoking doesn't mean you have to use a story about someone who smokes.

Take your time

Don't rush through your story, let the client enjoy it. When you have asked the client to do or imagine something in their head, pause to let them do it before moving on.

Humour

Jokes, puns, and comedy can add interest to a story, but people's sense of humour can be unpredictable, so use them with care and respect.

Tone and volume

You may use a calm or monotonous voice to get your clients into a trance or even just a relaxed state to prepare them for the metaphor. But once you get to the story, say it with expression. Vary your tone, speed, and volume to reflect what you're saying. If the story's exciting, sound excited, and so on.

Involve the client

Use words like imagine, think about, remember, consider, and not just visualise. Not all of us see internal images. (You'll find more detailed tips on dealing with non-visual clients in my book *The Hypnotherapist's Companion*.)

Ask questions, like 'What do you think happened then?' or attract their interest with comments like 'You will never guess what happened next'.

Don't be too obvious

There are two ways of delivering metaphors, one is to simply tell the tale and let them draw their own conclusions. The other is to end with something like 'And that is just like your situation because ...' You may feel explanations are needed but remember that one point of using metaphors is to avoid the client using conscious reasoning. You could always ask the client later what they thought of the story or why they thought you chose it.

Familiarity breeds confidence, not contempt

You certainly don't need to memorise all the stories in this book, or others. But you do need a certain familiarity with the story you're going to use with a client. Read it through a couple of times before your session, perhaps out loud.

Many of the metaphors and stories include *italics*. These are not intended to be read to your client. They are instructions to you, or they tell you to insert information about your client, (Make sure you have the relevant information before you begin.)

MAKING METAPHORS OF YOUR OWN

AUTHOR: DEBBIE WALLER

Inside each of us is a natural-born storyteller, waiting to be released.

Robin Moore, author[1]

I hope you will be inspired by this book to create some metaphors of your own, but some of you may be wondering if you can.

Let's face it, not everyone believes themselves to be a natural storyteller. (Or according to the quote above, perhaps they feel their inner storyteller is still firmly under lock and key!) Not everyone has a vast poetic vocabulary.

It doesn't matter.

When I got married, we chose to use the 'modern' form of language in our ceremony. (It was well before anyone considered writing their own vows, you only had the choice between archaic and modern). There is a power in traditional phrases like 'let no man put asunder' but we felt it was more meaningful to use the language we spoke every day when we made those promises to one another.

In the same way, the words you use when you tell stories can have the perfect meaning for your client no matter what style of language you use to present them.

Some of the stories in this book are multi-layered and have a certain complexity of language. But others use more straightforward and familiar ideas, words and phrases: check out the mini metaphors, for example.

So, give it a go. The joy of metaphors is that all approaches are equally powerful.

Tips for making your own metaphors

Help the client to identify with the protagonist by making them similar in some way. Ensure that, by the end, the protagonist learns a lesson, finds new strength, or makes a change that is relevant to the client's situation.

Use engaging, emotional and poetic language. Walking down a flight of stairs is not as engaging as floating or drifting down them.

Bill Cook[2] says when structuring your story, you should work with the acronym STORI, which stands for

- Set the scene – that could be 'What you said reminded me of ...' or (with older clients) 'Are you sitting comfortably? Then I'll begin ...' which opened every episode of *Listen with Mother,* a story-based children's radio programme on the BBC.
- Tell the listener about the problem – introduce your characters and setting, then describe the challenge the protagonist is facing.
- Organise a search for helpful resources – this tends to be the 'adventure' or 'journey' part of the story.
- Refine the therapeutic intervention – show how the protagonist learns to use the new resources to resolve the problem or show what goes wrong when they don't.

- Integrate the lesson – end the story by letting the main character clarify and perhaps describe the lesson or changes they experienced, and how this helped them.

Cook was working with children, but the principles apply equally well to therapeutic stories. After all, the point is that stories are used in this way because they appeal to the child within us all.

USING THE STORIES
IN THIS BOOK

AUTHOR: DEBBIE WALLER

As we've said, the ready-made stories in this book can be used as they are, but it will be better if they are tweaked to reflect something about your client and make it feel as if they were created just for them.

We'll give you some tips on personalising the stories as we go, but you can use your imagination and your own responses to them as well. If you don't have the book with you in the session, that's fine. What you remember of the story, combined with some ideas of your own, will be everything you need.

Another thing to note. Some of the stories have been written by hypnotherapists, who tend to use a trance induction before a metaphor. Because of this, several of them start with wording that implies the client is in a state of relaxation before getting to the nitty gritty.

If you are a counsellor, meditation teacher, or coach and don't use trance, I'd suggest beginning each one with a few relaxing breaths, or something like:

As you listen to this story, you'll probably start to relax and focus on the characters, places or situations involved. You might even choose to close your eyes to concentrate better, and that's fine.

Your interpretation of the story will be the right one and, the more you focus on it, the clearer its meaning will become, whether you consciously realise it or not....

Or, of course, if you're using them conversationally, feel free to omit any references to relaxation and jump straight in there with the story.

CHAPTER TWO

KALEIDOSCOPE: A TWIST ON SOME CLASSICS

There is no such thing as a new idea. It is impossible. We simply take a lot of old ideas and put them into a sort of mental kaleidoscope. We give them a turn and they make new and curious combinations.

Mark Twain[1]

We've already talked about how fairy stories change over time to suit both the storyteller and their audience (See the article Telling Stories at the beginning of this book for more). And, of course, this is also true of therapeutic tales. Think about 'The Control Room' for example. A simple idea of a room, containing lots of controls. Within the metaphor, the room stands for the client's unconscious, and the controls allow them to turn positive attributes like confidence higher, and negative ones like worry lower. But each therapist tells it differently, and each client responds to a different type of room. In fact, it's not even necessary that it is a room.

Someone who likes steampunk, for example, might enjoy building a machine with clockwork controls and a steam engine to make it work. A computer whizz might relate to going inside the motherboard of their mind and rewiring the connections. Fans of fantasy fiction might like to learn magic spells to alter the settings. And so on.

In fact, you'll see notes with each of the metaphors in this book, encouraging you to personalise them, and offering suggestions about how to adapt them to the client in front of you, and I'd encourage you to do just that.

However, in this chapter, we've given you a start. We have taken some familiar ideas and made our own 'new and curious combinations'. Each one draws on tradition but is undeniably special and unique.

Enjoy them, and hopefully take inspiration to create your own.

AROMAS AND RHYTHMS

AUTHOR: LARA MCCLURE

Personalisation:

A client's peaceful place is most often a natural environment where nothing much is happening – a forest, field or beach. Now and then, people choose a room in their home, and I heard Roy Hunter say at a conference that, when working with terminally ill clients, many chose their childhood bedrooms. But some clients respond better to something completely different.

For example, I had one whose 'peaceful place' was Times Square at midnight on the Millennium. It wasn't exactly peaceful as it included a soundtrack of fireworks, singing and shouting, but he wanted to tap into the amazing feelings he had at that event. And why not?

Here, we have something different again. The following was included to show how different sensory processing preferences can be utilised to make an old idea feel new.

The staircase draws on the sense of smell and would particularly suit those who use aromatherapy or like flowers, since you can adjust the scents to include their favourites. It could also be a good alternative for those who don't find it easy to visualise since it works with other senses.

The peaceful place at the bottom is based on Gabrielle Roth's Five Rhythms sequence, which is a movement meditation drawn from *indigenous and shamanic traditions, among others. It's all about energy and suggests that moving the body helps to free the heart, mind, and inspiration. The five movements are Flowing, Staccato, Chaos, Lyrical, and Stillness, in that order. As you read it here, think about how you could adapt this idea to include the rhythms of other dances and traditions for a client who enjoyed these activities.*

You could, of course, use these separately as well as together.

Olfactory staircase deepener

You find yourself at the top of a staircase, with an old, heavy, wooden banister, which looks smooth and inviting to the touch; you reach out and place your hand on it, finding it warm under your fingers as you decide to climb down.

You climb down onto the first step, finding that the carpet beneath your feet is thick, and soft, and velvety, your feet really sink into it as you begin to descend.

And as you begin to descend, you catch a faint scent which grows stronger and clearer as you go further down. To begin with, it is fresh and light, with high notes of linen and citrus, yuzu, bergamot and hesperidic fruits, and the sweet tang of mint and lemon balm.

You step down onto the next step, and find the carpet feels deeper and softer than on the step above. With each step you descend, it grows deeper and thicker, more and more plush and luxurious.

As you step down, the scents that surround you become thicker and richer too, ripe and fruity now: barberry and blackcurrant, thickening and deepening, almond and sesame, oleaginous and deep.

Deeper still, you find floral scents, heady and intoxicating: magnolia, stocks, delicate anemone, bright fuchsia, goldenrod and bitter belladonna. They fill your senses as you climb further down, deeper and deeper.

Another step transports you into a flavoursome fusion of

herbals, savoury and green: vervain and tulsi and meaty rosemary, such sweet sorrel, as you descend still further.

Next come the spices, filling your nose, and your head, and your heart, with warmth and depth: cinnamon and star anise and cloves. The weight and heft of pepper. Deep; relaxing; delicious.

And, still, you descend, deeper and deeper.

Deeper still lie the woods and mosses, earthy forest scents: sticky pine and heavy sandalwood, rich and deep and velvety dark. You breathe them in so very deeply, and descend again, deeper and deeper.

Then deepest of all, you are wrapped in an all-pervasive musk of animal smells: ambergris and a hint of fox on a deep, dark night. The deepest smells you can register, gunpowder and cordite, the lowest notes in the symphony of scent, leather and suede and tobacco, deep and dark, soothing yet exciting, entrancing.

And, as you descend to the very last step, you are surrounded and enveloped by the all-encompassing, unmistakable, familiar and delectable aroma of coffee. Your favourite blend, freshly ground and bursting with flavour and all that energetic potential.

Five rhythm peaceful place

You walk a little distance from the bottom of the staircase, stepping across that deep velvety carpet, and come to a door. You somehow know that you have come to the right place. With a smile spreading across your face, you grip the handle and open the door, which swings open easily to reveal a sunlit meadow.

Stepping through the door, you are aware of the warm sun on your back and a light breeze riffling through your hair. You step out onto the grass, soft and springy beneath your feet. You feel comfortable, relaxed, and happy to be here, and you pause at that moment. You have a feeling that you have arrived at last.

You become aware of music, faintly reaching you from across the meadow – a soft lilt of flowing notes, faint but sweet. Instinctively, you begin to move across the meadow towards it. You allow your body to move, gently and easily, finding yourself moving forwards in an elegant, languid surge, your body graceful and light, your movement rhythmic, fluid, flexible. You are travelling, but you are also dancing, you are flowing across the meadow.

You can trust your feet to travel to exactly where they need to be. The music grows more audible as you move towards the source of the sound and, as you do so, you become aware of other dancers, a positive and welcome presence of others, coming to your attention now as you flow towards them and feel their energy growing closer.

And, gradually, your movement expands and solidifies into more deliberate forms, percussive steps, growing more powerful and stronger as you begin to decide where to place each foot in a building structure of increasingly staccato rhythm. The other dancers are closer now, and their movements, too, are taking on a clearer structure, just like yours, as the music becomes louder and more insistent, compelling, enveloping,

Gradually that staccato rhythm builds, strengthens, and grows, wider and wilder, until all at once it bursts out of that structure into a spontaneous release of exuberant, chaotic JOY! You hear it in the increased intensity of the music, you feel it in the movements of your own body which becomes enormous, you seem somehow to fill the entire meadow. Your energy grows, reaches out and connects with the same energy pouring out of the other dancers, you are fully aware of their presence now, and it is welcome, joyful, and exhilarating.

Alongside and amongst them, you are liberated, you are released, and you are dizzyingly, wonderfully FREE! You experience a feeling of true physical abandon, glorious chaos, nothing holds you back as you surrender to the wild, exaggerated movements your body wants to make, twisting and gyrating and pulsing, burning with pure energy!

Until, inevitably, and at just the right moment, that great energy gradually begins to ebb and subside, your movements regulate and reduce in size. The music retreats to a calmer, softer, pulse. And your body returns to a more measured, elegant, pace, a more harmonious pattern, slowing and becoming lyrical, soulful, dignified, swaying and weaving,

And the movements of the other dancers mirror yours, their gentler, more lyrical shapes complement and tessellate with your own; together you progressively slow to a stately, regular rhythm, and that regularity of movement takes on a dream-like pace with space for reflection and stillness, your movements become smaller and more personal, your body draws in closer, you feel closer to your heart, closer to your soul, drawing inwards and downwards as you gradually sway to a soft stillness.

You feel deeply relaxed, perhaps more than you have for a long time. You feel refreshed and renewed. You feel free, and yet connected to the other dancers who have shared this space with you. You can sense that they, too, have drawn inwards, and are still. You have all the space you need, but you are not alone.

And this place in which you have enjoyed such wonderful movement and such profound connection is yours to access whenever you wish. All you need to do to get there is to close your eyes, find that staircase and climb down through the symphony of scents to the door.

The Author:

Lara McClure came to hypnotherapy through storytelling, and her practice is strongly rooted in that craft, finding profound therapeutic potential in carefully constructed bespoke narratives. Lara enjoys creating unique thoughtscapes to help individuals make positive changes in their lives. She loves a good metaphor as a creative and non-confrontational way to approach an issue sideways, which the subconscious mind instinctively 'gets'!

Lara is passionate about the evidence basis for her work and will often direct clients to scientific papers supporting the techniques used in their therapy. She teaches research methodology to students of acupuncture and Chinese Herbal

Medicine at the Northern College of Acupuncture in York, and loves how judicious use of evidence can support therapeutic decision-making and enhance the credibility of Complementary Therapies, an irresistible balance of science and art.

Lara is a mum to three and a Nana to two (so far!). She currently practises hypnotherapy in Pocklington, North Yorkshire in a multidisciplinary practice alongside acupuncturists and bodyworkers

- https://www.learntoheal.uk/team/lara-mcclure

HOT AIR BALLOON

AUTHOR: KATHLEEN ROBERTS

Personalisation:

There's a lot you can do with a metaphorical balloon. You can tie unwanted stuff to it and watch it float away, blow unwanted thoughts and feelings into it, release it, pop it, and lots more.

This take on the theme uses a hot air balloon, and the author says it was inspired by a client who described herself as 'feeling she had no control', 'bogged down', 'lost', 'panicking' and unable to gain any perspective. She wanted help with stress and anxiety and, although not having panic attacks, felt that if she carried on along her current trajectory, she might end up experiencing them. Some of her words and phrases appear in the script (for example, 'confusing', 'in control', 'oppressive thoughts' 'heart pounding') but you can swap them out for the words that your client uses.

Always check for height or flying phobias before using this one!

You are walking along a path in a woodland. There are trees all around you, they seem quite tall, crowding in, blocking out the light.

The path is bordered by dense vegetation; bushes and scrub

that hide the spaces between trees, and brambles that have grown across the path, making it difficult to walk easily. It's hard to see very far ahead, the path twists and turns, and everything feels as if it's closing in on you.

You've been walking along this path for a while now. It feels like a long time; you've no idea how far the wood stretches, but it must be enormous. It's a huge forest, it must go on for miles. You realise now that you're not sure of your bearings, or how to find your way home.

The forest is all around; it's all a confusing mass of undergrowth, dense thicket, and those tall trees that tower over you. The light is too dim to see properly, because it's dark under the canopy of woodland, even though it's daytime.

You can only catch a glimpse of the sky now and again, when the trees thin out a little, and then they crowd in again. And the path itself is narrow, sometimes it almost disappears, where the undergrowth and brambles have grown over it.

You feel oppressed amid all this woodland, not really knowing if you're going the right way, and you begin to feel your unease growing. And then comes the realisation that you're lost in the forest now, with no idea which way to go.

Your heart is beating faster, it's really pounding now. You're walking more quickly; strange noises are coming from the dense thickets on either side.

You feel you're about to panic, but there's no point in running, because you don't know which way to go. You're beginning to lose control.

And then, then ...

You tell yourself to stop it now, STOP.

You're going to take three, deep, breaths.

You stop walking, simply stop on the path and let your shoulders drop, let your body relax, and take the first breath, inhaling slowly, and then exhaling.

And then the next, and now, you feel your heart slowing down. Your mind clears.

And as you take in the third breath, that clarity increases, and you're feeling even more relaxed now, and as you exhale, letting go of the last bit of fear.

As you let that breath go, you retain within you that sense of calm, certainty, and you become aware that the sunlight is filtering through the trees. The noises in the wood are simply birdsong, a fresh breeze is ruffling your hair, and you can see bluebells in the glades by the side of the path, which now is smooth and clear and easy.

You take a confident step forward on that grassy, even path, and then you're walking ahead, purposefully. The trees are thinning out, the path widens, there's more brightness ahead, and suddenly you're in a forest clearing, wide and spacious, with plenty of light, and short green grass.

In the middle of the clearing is a hot air balloon, its canopy brightly striped, with a lovely wicker basket on the ground, sturdy and safe, roomy and solid. And, in the basket, is a man who is looking straight at you, smiling, cheerful, now he's waving, beckoning to you.

The sun is shining into the clearing, you can see that there are wildflowers in the grass, and the birds are singing their hearts out. You smile back at the cheery man and walk towards the balloon; you've always wanted to go on a balloon ride.

'Want a lift home?' he calls. 'Or is there anywhere else you fancy going?'

He takes your hand and helps you into the basket. You look around it and see there's a soft woolly blanket, a flask with a hot drink, and various little comforts for the ride.

The man is smiling at you. 'Ready for take-off?' he asks.

'Definitely,' you say. You're smiling.

And, with that, the balloon begins to rise gently, and you feel safe and secure; the man in charge of the balloon is clearly very competent. He smiles at you, and you feel a sense of delight and happy anticipation.

'Off we go,' he says. 'Everything looks much better from above.'

You smile back and feel that you've met a new friend, and then your new friend adds: 'We need to get some distance. Then you'll be able to see. Really see.'

The balloon soars gently and slowly above the clearing, not very high, but high enough so that you can look down at the landscape. You can see it spread out underneath you, like a contour map.

And, straight away, you're surprised because the forest isn't vast at all. What you can see from above is that, really, it's just a little wood, and you realise that you've been wandering round and round in circles, for a long time now, getting confused.

There are the trees below you, quite a few of them, but not enough to really get lost in, not if you stay calm. From above, they look quite small trees too, with plenty of open glades and woodland clearings.

What you thought was a huge forest is just a bit of woodland, in the middle of the countryside.

And not very far away is a town, or maybe a village, and then another village, lots of roads and even a railway line, and you can see rivers and streams, fields and farms. It's all ordinary and familiar, and suddenly you know just where everything is, you can place it on the map.

In a few minutes, you'll be able to see your house quite clearly. You can look down on the roof, the garden, and all the familiar things out there.

You think how silly you've been, you feel a bit embarrassed, and you look at the man and see that he's chuckling, he knows just what you're thinking.

'It's not your fault,' he says. 'When you're down there, in the middle of it all, you really can't see the wood for the trees.' And you laugh out loud at this, it sounds so ridiculous.

And a little while later, when the ride is over and you're walking up to your own front door, you can turn and wave at the new friend in the balloon, and he waves back, as he soars up into the air again.

Perhaps he's going to look for someone else who needs to gain some distance, some perspective.

But it's a revelation, that you really couldn't see the wood for the trees, and that vast forest that seemed so sinister is now just a place where you might walk a dog for ten minutes, or go for a short stroll with friends, or take a picnic.

And you see now that perspective is everything, gaining some distance, not being down amongst the undergrowth and the scrub that's stopping you from seeing where you are, but rising above that, so that you can see more accurately.

Getting some distance is what it's all about, that's the key, whether it's

[*Replace the next paragraph with examples that are personal to your client.*]

getting some help from a friend, getting away from the problems that are oppressing you, or just relaxing for a while, meditating, doing something enjoyable, or grounding yourself in deep breathing.

And, suddenly, that perspective is there, you can see quite clearly: you can focus, solve problems, and be resourceful and creative, once you have perspective.

And now you've learned to gain some distance, to have perspective, and you will never be lost in the forest again.

You can take three deep breaths, rise above the oppressive thoughts, look down at the problems, and once you're up there, looking down, they are smaller than you thought, more manageable. Perhaps some are even insignificant, and with that perfect calmness and clarity, you can take control.

The Author:

Kathleen Roberts is a former journalist, lecturer and local authority officer. She trained as a hypnotherapist with Yorkshire Hypnotherapy Training and is now one of their independent assessors. She also works as an educational consultant and is one of a panel of expert assessors for the EU's Erasmus+ scheme.

THE RAINCOAT

AUTHOR: DEBBIE WALLER

Personalisation:

T his is a variation on the theme of the 'Protective Bubble' metaphor, with which I am sure you are familiar. Essentially, you ask the client to imagine a shield or bubble which completely protects them from all the challenges of life. Good things are kept close; not-so-good ones bounce off so they can be seen from a different perspective, as smaller and less troublesome, and dealt with appropriately more easily.

I would generally use this for clients living in ongoing stressful environments, for example, if they have a nightmare boss or difficult family situation. But it's also useful for shorter-term issues, such as dealing with a Christmas visit from a critical family member.

You can make the shield or bubble anything you feel your client will relate to. Literally a shield or even armour for those who like role play games or fantasy fiction, a magical Patronus for those who enjoy the adventures of a certain boy wizard, an apron for those who like cooking, and so on. But this one takes us back to those times when all your clothes were bought too big on the theory that you'd 'grow into it'. We've all been there.

Adapt this to suit by using boy instead of girl if you are a male *therapist and making the coat the client's favourite colour if you know what that is.*

Someone said to me the other day that troubles are like rain. You put up with a few drops because, although you get a bit wet, it's not enough to really notice.

But then, if the rain keeps on falling you do start to notice, and to get wetter and wetter, and then you really can't think about anything except how wet and uncomfortable you are, until you come up with a good way to keep dry.

It got me thinking about this raincoat I had when I was a little girl. My Mum always bought my coats too big, so I could grow into them, and this one came right down over the tops of my boots. The arms were so long that my hands were right up inside the sleeves, and the hood was so big it covered my whole face, so I could hardly see out.

It was bright red and made of plastic, and I loved it. I felt safe and warm and protected there inside it, and so happy that nothing bothered me.

I used to splash around, and I didn't care whether there were just a few drops of rain or a downpour. I think someone could have thrown a whole bucket of water over me in that coat and I would still have stayed dry.

I felt so safe and protected in that coat, because the rain would just run off me. The coat was so long that it even kept my feet dry – the water just trickled off it and onto the floor, and then it flowed away from me, and soaked into the ground to help beautiful flowers grow.

Maybe you can see it now in your mind's eye, that little girl splashing around in the rain in a bright red raincoat.

And next time it rains on you, you can imagine how it felt to be inside that coat, feeling safe and warm and happy, despite the rain that was falling, just waiting it out till the flowers start to grow.

The Author:

Debbie Waller is a hypnotherapist in Normanton, West Yorkshire. She is also a hypnotherapy supervisor and Director/Head Tutor of Yorkshire Hypnotherapy Training. She is the author of 'Their Worlds, Your Words', and 'The Hypnotherapist's Companion', a contributor to the 'Hypnotherapy Handbook' and past editor of the 'Hypnotherapy Journal'. And, of course, contributing editor of this book of metaphors.

SARAH'S TRAVELS
AUTHOR: LARA MCCLURE

Personalisation:

*T*ravel metaphors are tried and tested, often reflecting the client's life journey. This is a great example of how a very traditional approach can be adapted to a very modern issue; social media addiction and FOMO (Fear of Missing Out).

To help the client identify with Sarah, you could change her name or gender, or add a few details that make her more like the client – a distinctive brooch or red hair, for example.

Although this is aimed at social media addiction, with a few appropriate tweaks, it could also be used for clients who are unable to settle on anything, those who never quite complete a task because they are always distracted by the 'next big thing', or those who feel they are constantly busy but achieving nothing.

Sarah loved to travel. At every opportunity, she would jet off to horizons new, always seeking a fresh experience, different landscapes and faces. She loved to leap onto planes, jump aboard trains, or climb into her car, spontaneously and joyfully, and see where she might end up. All her free time and holidays were spent in this way, jetting everywhere in a whirlwind – it was an exciting approach to life and an amazing way to connect with people.

In fact, Sarah hardly felt alive at all in the times in between her frequent trips, itching to be off again and impatient with the inertia she felt when she wasn't on the move. As a result, when she did get the chance to get away, she moved as fast as she could to fit as much as possible into the time she had. Between trips, she felt caged, tethered, disconnected.

Eventually, Sarah felt that she needed to be on the move literally all the time, seeking out new places, novel sights, higher mountains, and wider horizons. She felt an inescapable urge to go to more and more locations at an ever more frenetic pace to maximise the use of her time. Each place she went offered connections to other, newer destinations, further away, and Sarah felt compelled to follow each trail. She spent less and less time in each place she visited, noticed fewer and fewer details, and retained only fleeting impressions of where she had been – and of the ever-increasing numbers of people she encountered there.

Sarah was afraid that if she stopped moving, she would miss something important. Someone else might see something she hadn't seen, hear something she had yet to hear, visit a place that Sarah herself had never been to. So she kept going. She was spending all her time moving, moving, moving, on a constant quest with no real end goal, which felt like it had no way of ending.

Sarah's restlessness was getting in the way of the rest of her life. When she saw her friends, she was always on her way somewhere else, so she hardly took the time to meet anyone's eye. Although, in theory, she had met and connected with thousands of people, deep down Sarah felt like she didn't know any of them very well, and she doubted if any of them knew her any better. Her relationships felt brittle, shallow, and transient.

Sarah realised that because she never stopped moving, she was missing everything.

So, one day, Sarah tried something that felt risky and brave; she stood still for a moment.

It was difficult at first, the desire to dash off in one direction or another was overwhelmingly strong, but, as Sarah stayed in one place, she noticed features of the world around her that overcame that restlessness. She saw the colours of the buildings, and the clothes of passers-by. She heard the noises of the city in the early morning; a distant cathedral bell; a hum of traffic; snatches of conversation; a dog barking. Each new facet of the world that unfolded around her revealed itself, one by one, as she calmly stayed where she was and took notice of what was around her. She caught the scent of flowers from the stall by the station, and rich, dense coffee smells escaping from the little kiosk there. Her mouth began to water at the idea of stopping there for a cinnamon bun. She felt the firmness of the ground beneath her feet, and a slight breeze riffling through her hair. Sarah felt elated, liberated, *alive*.

At that moment, Sarah resolved to move more slowly, to pay more attention, and to enjoy the process of being somewhere without rushing to leave it behind. Her ability to concentrate gradually began to build. She focused on a smaller number of locations, a tighter circle of closer connections to people she really cared about, and who cared about her.

Sarah still travels, though at a statelier pace, and with a new sense of genuine connectedness to the worlds through which she moves – and the people in them. Quality has triumphed over quantity in Sarah's travels, in her relationships and in her journey through life.

The Author:

Lara McClure came to hypnotherapy through storytelling, and her practice is strongly rooted in that craft, finding profound therapeutic potential in carefully constructed bespoke narratives. Lara enjoys creating unique thoughtscapes to help individuals make positive changes in their lives. She loves a good metaphor as a creative and non-confrontational way to approach an issue sideways, which the subconscious mind instinctively 'gets'!

Lara is passionate about the evidence basis for her work and will often direct clients to scientific papers supporting the techniques used in their therapy. She teaches research methodology to students of acupuncture and Chinese Herbal Medicine at the Northern College of Acupuncture in York, and loves how judicious use of evidence can support therapeutic decision-making, and enhance the credibility of Complementary Therapies, an irresistible balance of science and art.

Lara is a mum to three and a Nana to two (so far!). She currently practises hypnotherapy in Pocklington, North Yorkshire in a multidisciplinary practice alongside acupuncturists and bodyworkers

- https://www.learntoheal.uk/team/lara-mcclure.

CHAPTER THREE

FINDING INNER STRENGTH AND RESILIENCE

I recall a client who came to me with a public speaking phobia. When I asked about his hobbies, he told me he was the chairman of his local golf club. I asked how he managed at the Annual General Meeting, and he looked at me blankly, not realising that he was, in fact, already a confident public speaker. Apparently, it was just work that was the problem!

This is an example of a client who didn't recognise that he had the strengths and resources he wanted, he just needed to reinforce them and transfer them to a new situation. You also find situations where clients haven't used their skills for a while, and have almost forgotten they have them, and still others where clients need new skills built from scratch.

In this chapter, you'll find metaphors that encourage them to do all those things. To build or rebuild, discover or rediscover the inner strengths and power that they need to achieve their goals.

It's best to follow any of these with some future pacing – ask the client to imagine themselves in the future, using their new resources effectively and feeling amazing. Allow them to compare how good this feels with what they would have previously experienced in those situations, so they will never want to go back. And always end the session on a high, reinforcing their confidence in their new abilities, feelings, or behaviours.

THE ASTRONAUT

AUTHOR: STEVE LOVATT

Personalisation:

T he following was originally developed for clients who were reporting increased anxiety regarding the end of the various COVID 19 lockdowns, expressing an intense fear of an unknown future, but you can use it to support those who present with anxiety around all kinds of unknown events and experiences. It reframes and normalises their anxiety responses and allows them to move through them to a calmer place.

It is based on the idea of early space travel, which few have experienced, but many have witnessed. For this reason, the author says it appears to resonate particularly well with those clients who have a living memory of this time. You can include references to specific friends or family who offer support where appropriate – placing them as companions in the capsule, in the thoughts of the astronaut contemplating Mother Earth and/or waiting on the ship on the return home.

It is not advisable to use this script with clients who experience claustrophobia, fear of water, or fear of heights, due to the nature of the imagery and metaphors used.

.   .   .

Sitting there completely calm, completely relaxed, I'd like you to imagine you're about to begin an amazing, exciting journey. Maybe you can imagine adventures that you've been on before, or maybe adventures you've dreamed of having – remembering that tingling expectation in your tummy.

As you imagine this adventure, you may begin to realise just how vivid your imagination can be, either as vivid photographs, detailed, colourful, and in focus. Or maybe amazing pictures or art drawn or painted by skilled artists with a vast, limitless array of paints, pencils, brushes, and colours. Or maybe listening to a detailed story written by a skilled author.

I am going to take you on a journey, a story and you can allow your amazing imagination to paint pictures, take photos, or weave stories around it, adding details from your own experiences or imagination. Knowing that you are in the right place, at the right time, with nothing to do, and nowhere to go, completely safe and sound. All you need to do is listen to the sound of my voice.

Imagine that you are an astronaut, an astronaut in the early days of manned space flight, supported by all the brilliant brains at NASA. Imagine the rigorous training you have completed, the hours of training and testing, the checks and rechecks, the health checks, the technical checks, and the equipment checks. Now feeling confident, safe, and relaxed.

Imagine that today is the day, your day, your first day in space. It's quite natural to notice some trepidation, maybe feeling the next few moments, seconds, minutes, or hours are unknown. But – what you do know is that all the preparations have been made, everything has been double-checked, triple-checked.

All the experts agree. You are prepared. They are prepared. You are ready for an adventure.

Your adventure.

You climb into your space capsule, making yourself comfortable, safe and secure. Your companions are there with you, as the final checks are made. All the safety checks are in place, as the capsule's door is closed.

You feel the oxygen supply in your helmet as it enters your lungs, noticing the natural flow of your breath, allowing yourself to breathe naturally, calmly. Noticing, as you inhale, how your belly rises and how, as you exhale, your belly falls. Just following the natural, calm, safe, relaxing breath. Allowing any tension to gently subside, to be replaced by a feeling of adventurous anticipation.

This is your first space flight and, although you have trained, and spoken to skilled and experienced people who have been in space before, you cannot help but feel a little anxiety, but you know this is normal. You know this is what it feels like to be excited, it's not unexpected or something to be worried about.

As you sit in the capsule you hear the countdown,

[*Count down very slowly, timing the numbers with the client's out breath.*]

10, 9, 8, 7, 6, 5, 4, 3, 2, 1.

And then you feel the surge of adrenalin as your whole body, all your senses, experience the excitement of the launch. Maybe feeling a little fear, a little anxiety, but knowing this is normal and will soon pass. Focussing your mind on what is happening right now, the things you need to do. Accept that anxiety is a natural coping mechanism, to keep us aware and ready to react, but know that once the initial feeling subsides, so will the anxiety. It's normal and natural to feel anxious sometimes, everyone does.

And then the engines quieten, and you find yourself in a place of sublime calmness, of weightlessness, without a weight or care on your mind, a time for rest and relaxation, a time to move away from anxiety.

You realise that the anxiety you felt earlier was to be expected, not to be feared. And you also recognise that that time has now passed, and you feel your body relaxing, your breathing becoming calm, your heart rate slowing, and even those butterflies in your tummy now seem quiet.

You notice the Earth through one of the windows, Mother Earth, home. Maybe you have spiritual thoughts or maybe your thoughts turn to nature and our beautiful, small, blue planet. Earth. Allow your mind a few moments of quiet contemplation.

[*Pause.*]

Your mind now begins to think of the adventure which has only just begun, how maybe things might be different, how you may be different when you return to Earth.

You feel a strong sensation of optimism, an understanding that many things change. It's normal to feel anxious about change, but change is the natural flow of life. You realise that the very spice of life, of any adventure, can be found in the unknown, and the unknown is nothing to be fearful of. Allow this realisation, this wisdom, to be absorbed into every muscle, bone, tendon, ligament, and organ, into every cell of your body.

[*Pause.*]

Now, it's time to return, to go back to Earth, back home. Although, perhaps, you feel strongly comfortable in this calm place, this safe place, you know you must return. Return to a world which may feel very different, but you have confidence that it will be good to get back home, great to be back to normality, whatever that new normal may feel like. You know that life continues, and you have all you need to navigate your journey, all the knowledge, experience, wisdom, love, and support you need.

So, tighten your safety belt and begin your descent back to Earth. Maybe, at times, that readjustment might seem a little rocky, a little loud, a little disorientating, and a little overwhelming. But you recall that initial lift-off. How feelings of trepidation and anxiety are normal and will pass sooner than you think.

Soon they do pass, and you find yourself drifting back to earth. From the darkness of space to a beautiful blue sky, and then you feel the support of the parachutes as they open and gently lower you back through wispy white clouds, drifting down, until you gently splash down into a crystal blue sea.

The journey, the adventure, is completed, and this small moment in time has taught you so much.

How to accept anxiety as natural at times, and how to travel through it. How often to give yourself permission to re-engage that sense of calmness and relaxation. and to release yourself from anxiety when it's no longer needed. How to have faith in preparation, to allow others to support and guide you. How to appreciate the gift of life, our wonderful home, this planet Earth.

As the support crew opens the door to the capsule and takes you to a waiting ship, you see friends, family, and loved ones waiting. You wonder what might have changed, and you realise we all experience change, it's part of life. You think back to the other historic moments in your life, maybe when famous people or royalty have passed, weddings, births, changes in your job, your home, your relationships.

You feel that this journey has taught you so many things, and so much wisdom has been shared with you. The greatest are that anxiety will pass, and the gift of calmness and relaxation, relaxing away from the anxious state.

You feel fully equipped to embrace change, to enjoy the continuing adventure, the opportunity of change, with calmness and confidence.

The Author:

Steve Lovatt is a holistic hypnotherapist, Soma breath coach, Theta healer, dream yoga facilitator, mindfulness practitioner, mindful meditation practitioner, and sound therapist. Working from his private practice at the edge of the Yorkshire Dales, he has a particular interest in anxiety and trauma release, using a tapestry of modalities to guide through healing pathways, using a journey of discovery within the subconscious mind. He also is a lecturer for a national training provider, training therapists in the areas of anxiety release, trauma, PTSD, and CPTSD. He works with several corporate clients, using his extensive corporate experience to assist them in their staff wellbeing programmes. Steve's website can be found at www.yourtimewellness.uk.

FAITH IN FIVE

AUTHOR: CHRISTINE HOWSON

Personalisation:

The aim of this script is generic, and it can be modified for use with a variety of issues, from panic attacks to general anxiety. It may be more of a guided meditation than a metaphor, strictly speaking, combining the 5-4-3-2-1 anti-anxiety technique (based on the five physical senses) with spiritual ideas. But this allows the unconscious mind to work positively with the spiritual one and provides a powerful impetus for change.

Faith is an area from which people draw much strength, but it must be used carefully and respectfully in therapy. As a practising Catholic, the author has used Christian-based religious suggestions for the first set of suggestions for each sense, and more nature-based ones for the second. However, these can be modified for all types of faith sources as you and your client see fit.

Before using this metaphor, ensure:

- *You have discussed and understood your client's beliefs and reassured them that you will use these ethically.*
- *The place and type of worship you include has positive or neutral associations for your client.*

The following assumes you have established ideomotor responses (finger or hand movements to indicate yes and no) before beginning. But if you don't generally use these, you can simply ask for a nod instead. As there is quite a lot of interaction, and multiple options in the way responses are given, make sure you have read through the technique thoroughly before using it with a client. Adjust the parts of the script relating to senses as necessary for clients who are visually impaired, etc.

Take a breath in and let it out without any judgement. Just notice the way it enters and leaves your body. Now imagine you are breathing in and out, the breath given to you by your faith. Each in-breath you take brings you closer to your faith and each out-breath helps you to offer up to

[*state the name of their God/Faith source*]

Any obstacles, fear, shame or worry, named or without a name, that may be troubling or triggering you. Perhaps you have climbed steps to enter your

[*church or place of prayer*]

or perhaps you have journeyed to your favourite place in nature. Take a moment, now, to make that journey and when you are in your spiritual home just give me a yes signal.

[*Pause and wait for the sign.*]

Now, you are in this place, sitting there safe and secure, knowing that this is somewhere you can be open, honest, and shielded from all harm and danger. Totally safe and totally secure.

Every breath you take in this place is cleansing both your mind and body in the presence of

[*state the name of their God/Faith source.*]

Each breath, and the sound of my voice, is allowing you to relax more and more. To sink deeper and deeper into your faith and become more and more aware of your spirit. Safe and protected from harm by all the tenets of your faith and beliefs. Focus on *that presence* with each breath in and out saying aloud or silently and slowly with a quiet pause say the words '*Guide me*'.

One word, one breath, knowing that your call is heard, and you are not alone. Noticing, now, how your breathing is already steadying as it enters and leaves your body. Speaking calmly and respectfully in the presence of your faith. Uttering this prayer from your heart in the way you know. There is nothing but sincerity and the truth and understanding that you seek. Just repeat the word 'Guide' on the in-breath and 'me' on the out-breath. And then, having spoken, wait a moment for the answer, and give me a nod when you wish me to continue.

[*Pause and wait for the sign.*]

Now, take a deep breath and imagine that breath reaching down and filling your lungs with air, healing energy, and blessings. Hold it for a moment and then breathe out at your own pace, shedding doubts and worries, and relaxing you deeper and deeper as you exhale.

As you swap the movements of the breath, notice your body and how it feels without judgement or restraint. As you are sharing this moment with

[*state the name of their God/Faith source*]

you recognise that knowledge of being heard and comforted spreading throughout your body. Just give me a yes signal when you wish me to continue.

[*Pause and wait for the sign.*]

Supporting you now, as much as you need, is your helpful and powerful subconscious mind. It draws your attention to your senses. Senses that we all have, and yet so often take for granted. Now, in full mindfulness, as we count down from five to one using our senses gifted by

[*state the name of their God/Faith source.*]

You recognise the power of the senses gifted to you. If one or more senses are easier to identify than others, that's fine. There is no need to struggle but allow your powerful and helpful subconscious mind to find the answers you are searching for in your faith and belief system.

In a moment, we're going on a journey of the senses. So,

continue to breathe in and out, easily and naturally, at your pace. If you need me to help you at any time with suggestions, just raise a finger on your hand as we discussed, and I will offer suggestions for you. Or I will remain silent until you give me a signal to continue.

You can say what you perceive aloud or silently in your head and give me a nod or a sign when you're ready to move on. So, are you ready?

[*Pause and wait for their nod or yes signal, and then start the Five Senses Journey.*]

Imagine you are in a huge and holy place that's inspiring you with awe and wonder, whether it's familiar or recalled. Perhaps it's a cathedral or temple that is manmade. Or it could be a wonder of nature.

With the next in-breath now count five things that you can see, or love to see, created by

[*state the name of their God/Faith source.*]

then release the breath at your pace and continue to breathe in and out evenly. Say these five things aloud or in your head, then give me a nod when you're ready to move on or raise a finger if you need suggestions of what you might see.

[*Suggestions, if needed, might include*
stained glass windows, huge columns, altars, candles, statues,
trees, hills, valleys, lakes, seashores, canyons, rivers.
Continue when you have the five things or the nod.]

Now, with the next in-breath, count four things that you can hear, or love to hear, created by

[*state the name of their God/Faith source.*]

As you continue to breathe in and out evenly in your place of worship, say these four things aloud or silently in your head, then give me a nod when you're ready to move on or raise a finger if you need suggestions of what you might hear.

[*Suggestions, if needed, might include:*
organ music, hymns being sung, the sound of prayers, the words of
the community

bird song, wind rustling the leaves, sounds of the river, the ebb and flow of the sea.

Continue when you have the four things or the nod.]

Now, with the next in-breath, list three things that you can smell, or scents that you like, created by

[state the name of their God/Faith source.]

in this sacred space as you continue to breathe in and out evenly. Say these three things aloud or silently in your head, then give me a nod when you're ready to move on, or raise a finger if you need suggestions of things you might smell.

[Suggestions, if needed, might include:

incense, wood polish, the smell of candles

flowers, leaves, grass.

Continue when you have the three things or the nod.]

Now, with the next in-breath, count two things that you can touch or feel created by

[state the name of their God/Faith source]

as you continue to breathe in and out evenly. Say these two things aloud, or silently in your head, then give me a nod when you're ready to move on, or raise a finger if you need suggestions of things that you might touch or feel.

[Suggestions, if needed, might include:

feel of the seat beneath you, the hymn book, a candle in your hand

the bark of a tree, the softness of the grass, the delicacy of a flower's petals.

Continue when you have the two things or the nod.]

Now, with the next in-breath, identify one thing that you can taste, or recall tasting, created by

[state the name of their God/Faith source]

as you continue to breathe in and out evenly. Say this one thing aloud, or silently in your head, then give me a nod when you're ready to move on or raise a finger if you need suggestions of things you might taste.

[Suggestions, if needed, might include:

the taste of communion, a meal shared with fellow parishioners

*the taste of refreshing water, a picnic enjoyed in the open air, the taste
of the air.*

Continue when you have one thing, or the nod.]

Notice how you feel now. Your unconscious mind has relaxed
and already you are feeling calmer and more in control. If you need
to repeat the five senses journey, just do so, lingering longer on the
senses that are strongest for you. We are all gifted with different
talents or modalities from our creator and move in this universe in
our own unique way.

As you breathe easily and comfortably at your pace allow
yourself to relax, noting the swapping of the breath without
controlling it at all. Swapping the in-breath for the out-breath. The
out-breath for the in.

If you notice the sounds around you, just accept them and don't
try to suppress them. Contrast them with the quiet within you,
swap thoughts for awareness, awareness for thoughts.

Allow yourself, with each breath, to consider this wonderful
place of your faith, wherever that may be. A place that is safe and
secure, where you are comfortable, and where you feel deep
contentment surrounding you, filling you, as though sinking into
the most comfortable state of calm for body, mind and spirit.
Secure and safe in a deep calm. Giving up to

[state the name of their God/Faith source]

any worries and concerns you have carried with you to this
sacred place, feel them lifted from you one by one, breath by
breath, as you open your mind and heart, your spirit and inner
being to listen and receive.

[Pause.]

As you are wrapped in the love of this sacred space you feel very
relaxed, more relaxed than you have felt for a very long time.
Allowing your worries to drain away, draining away and not
returning to your body or mind or spirit.

You feel these thoughts leaving you and being replaced by
feelings of comfort, kindness and compassion. A sense of deep
contentment fills you and the certainty that you have within you, as

a creation of Divine blessings, all you need to match and meet the challenges that face you each day. More than match, in fact – to overcome them and thrive in the challenges of each day. This sense of deep happiness is rooted in each of your five senses with great certainty, and it comes to the surface of your mind, making you smile.

You recall a film you saw of a visit you made to your sacred place. You saw how you entered in desperation and sought guidance and help. You see how by using your five senses of sight, sound, smell, touch, and taste, how you were wrapped up in the comfort of your faith and given great strength and all the resources you needed. Given more than you had ever asked.

When you can see this, just give me a nod or a sign.

[*Wait for the nod or sign.*]

That's good. Now see yourself counting down from five, four, three two, one – from sight, sound, smell, touch and taste, and being so unified with the presence of

[*state the name of their God/Faith source*]

that you notice clearly the differences in your facial expression, your body language, your breath.

When you can feel this, just give me a nod or a sign.

[*Wait for the nod or sign.*]

That is so good, Now see yourself receiving the support you asked for without words or any need to question. Just receiving because you asked and, as you asked you received, so you see how much more positive you look and how much happier you feel.

When you can notice this, just give me a nod or a sign.

[*Wait for the nod or sign.*]

Perhaps you can see yourself opening your palms outwards, and where, before, you were inward-looking, now you are outward-looking and looking around you. When you can see this, just give me a nod or a sign.

[*Wait for the nod or sign.*]

Perhaps now you are witnessing yourself listening and receiving the answers you asked for in your words of 'Guide me'. When you can see this, just give me a nod or a sign.

[*Wait for the nod or sign.*

NB: Whether a nod comes, or doesn't, after a while make the statement as follows:]

We know, as finite beings, that our timeframe and understanding are limited by their very definitions, but we also know that if we ask, we will receive, and that is the blessing of our faith.

Answers given today will stay with us and support us in the minutes, hours, days, weeks, and years ahead. Transforming, supporting, and helping us. Strengthening, motivating, and guiding us. Our timeframe is not that of

[*state the name of their God/Faith source*]

but by us being aware that we have received our answers and are ready to believe, knowing that we are blessed with them gives us huge strength.

So now it is time to leave this sacred place, but we know that, whenever it is safe for us to do so, we can find it again easily and immediately just by tapping into our senses and linking our needs with our spiritual journey.

The Author:

Christine Howson is a qualified, professional Hypnotherapist, Meditation Teacher and Mental Health First Aider providing NLP, coaching, mindfulness and meditation techniques.

She says: for me, every client is an important individual, and their therapy is matched specifically to their needs. Five-star Google reviews and fabulous testimonials make me very humble in being able to enable my clients to thrive. Working face-to-face in my therapy room, locally in Knaresborough and online, with clients aged from eight to over eighty, is a huge privilege. Inclusion is very important to me, so my clinics have disability access if needed. Flexibility is also imperative, to ensure each client receives the best bespoke service they deserve.

Being a former Modern Languages teacher, I can offer therapy in French and Spanish, and have even delivered relaxation therapy in Italian! I love the power of words and I am currently writing my own book, so please look out for it!

Perhaps my effective range of therapeutic strategies, along with the experience of having taught over 10,000 students, may be the heart of my success with clients? Above all, each client benefits from my expertise and knows they will be listened to non-judgementally and be treated with the respect and the highest professional care they deserve.

Claritas is Latin for clarity, and this is both the aim of my work and my practice name: clarity in thought and action. www.claritastherapy.com

FOOL'S GOLD

AUTHOR: SARAH LAMONT

Personalisation:

T his metaphor is presented as it was used for a weight reduction client, but it could be used for pretty much any presenting issue if you stick with the basic principles of

- *seeing themselves in the mirror after achieving their goals*
- *admiring their successful self and*
- *finding a note giving relevant affirmations.*

The 'Fool's Appetite' will change to 'Fool's Desire' (e.g., for cigarettes) or whatever else represents the temptation to return to the unwanted feeling, behaviour or habit.

[Take the client to their peaceful place. Then say:]
As you relax, allowing this sense of deep relaxation to continue, you suddenly become aware of a small path
[*use 'corridor' instead if the client's peaceful place is indoors*]
that you didn't notice before. A wave of curiosity comes over

you, and you may think, 'I wonder where that leads to?', so you begin to follow it. As you follow the path along,

[from outside] you notice a building ahead, there is a door.

[from inside] you move along the corridor, and as you turn a corner you notice a door.

Imagine you are standing in front of that door; walk right up to the door and notice the shape and the colour, the way it's set into the wall, the door handle and what that's like. Reach out your hand and take hold of the handle, noticing its texture and temperature against the palm of your hand. Use the door handle to open the door; it feels heavy, but it opens easily.

As you open the door and step through, you find yourself inside a room. It's the perfect temperature for you, and you feel safe and comfortable. The lighting is just how you like it, as you glance around the room noticing how it is furnished. Choose the colours of the walls, the texture of the floor under your feet, whether it is tiles, marble, or carpet, and whether you can hear your own footsteps as you move further into the room and begin to look around.

Amongst the furnishings, you notice that on one wall is the most beautiful mirror, covering the wall from floor to ceiling. It's a spotless and flawless mirror. You notice that it is reflecting the beauty of your room, and it also reflects your image, although your image is not quite clear, not quite in focus. As you look closer, you notice that the image is clearing, and the focus is beginning to sharpen. You are looking at yourself, but it is a slightly different you from the one you're used to seeing. As you look closer still, you realise that as the image becomes crystal clear, this is the most perfect self-image.

You are your ideal size and weight.

You have never been so happy to see your own image. You start to pose and admire your attractiveness, turning to the right, turning to the left, turning in such a way as to see your rear view. Every way you turn, it is you in the mirror, but a perfect you. You admire how perfectly shaped and proportioned you are, how your size and weight are perfectly balanced to your natural proportions. You are still you, but you look so good. You are a healthier, slimmer, shapelier, and more attractive you. And as you gaze upon the reflection in front of you, you enjoy knowing that this beautiful/handsome, attractive person is you.

[*Pause.*]

You now understand what you need to do, because you realise what you really look like, what you should look like, and what you deserve to look like when you do good things for yourself. Looking at yourself now, you realise how easy this is going to be, enjoying that version of yourself in that mirror now, you know how simple this is. Knowing that the reason you look so good, and feel so good, is the result of your respect and love for your own body. Looking in that mirror now, and seeing that image, is the result of your lifestyle changes, your balanced, healthy eating and exercise habits.

And looking at that image you realise you are already on your way to success. A success that is easy and enjoyable. A lifestyle change that will be with you now and for the rest of your life, because it is an easy and enjoyable way to live, and you know what the results will be like.

You happen to glance around the room and notice a table that you didn't see before. On that table is a piece of paper. Walk over to the table and pick it up.

The first thing that catches your eye is the writing, you recognise it as your own handwriting. 'Hang on a minute,' you think. 'I don't remember writing that'. But that doesn't matter.

All that matters is that you have written this, the self in the mirror has written it for you. So, you start to read.

First, it says: I eat only when I am physiologically hungry.

Now, look at the healthier, slimmer, more attractive you in the mirror. This message is from that image right there. The you, right there, that found it so easy and enjoyable to follow this message. To follow this guidance that you are now reading.

Next, it says: I enjoy drinking water and find that I need to drink a glass of water before I eat. Water is so cool and refreshing, I love the taste so much that I find myself much thirstier than I was previously.

Look at the image in the mirror again, that is you and you are now excited to follow the guidelines laid out in the note you have left on the table.

The next lines say: I eat and want only those foods that are good for my body. My stomach is smaller and getting smaller with every day that passes.

I eat mindfully; that is, I concentrate on one mouthful at a time, enjoying the food in my mouth rather than thinking about the next mouthful.

I enjoy tasting my food, eating more slowly means I eat less but enjoy it more.

I always leave food on my plate; this is not being disrespectful to the chef or wasteful. I just don't need it. I stop eating even before I am full, and I would rather it was put in the waste bin than on my waist.

I only eat what my body needs.

Look at the image again and remind yourself of why you are reading this note.

I exercise more. The more I exercise, the better I feel and the better I feel the more I exercise. I am always aware of how much exercise my body can handle and I ensure I keep to a level safe for me.

I look better and feel better day after day. My clothes are fitting loosely, and I feel good about myself.

I find myself smiling more and walking differently. Everyone notices how good I look.

I now have an abundance of confidence and my self-esteem has never been higher.

Look at your reflection in the mirror, see who you really are, know that this is easy and enjoyable, because if your reflection can do this, so can you. Say to your reflection, 'I am you and you are me, together we have achieved this.'

Take a long look at the healthier, slimmer, more attractive you in the mirror.

[*Pause.*]

You will have heard of Fool's Gold, because it resembles gold to the untrained eye. Prospectors used to collect it, hoping to sell it, only to be disappointed and frustrated that all their hard work had only resulted in something worthless. Fool's Appetite is just like Fool's Gold.

When you mistake appetite for a real bodily need, you end up frustrated and disappointed. Boredom is not hunger, frustration is not hunger, disappointment is not hunger, loneliness is not hunger, and worry is not hunger.

These feelings will never be resolved by eating food. They are Fool's Appetite, and you are no fool.

Looking in that mirror, at the healthier, slimmer, more attractive you, proves that you are not a fool. You are a beautiful, perfect, one-of-a-kind individual with an abundance of confidence and self-esteem which allows you to overcome all sorts of challenges in your life. You know that Fool's Appetite cannot be satisfied with food, because it's not real hunger. The image in that mirror is real, your determination to achieve any goal is real, and your confidence is real. You are that image, see who you really are through that image, you know that this is easy and enjoyable, because you have already achieved it.

You notice that you are smiling more and more, you feel more and more confident because you feel so good about yourself, and what you continue to achieve. You are living a healthier lifestyle that allows you to eat only when you are physiologically hungry, enjoy drinking water, only eat and want foods that are good for you, eat mindfully, tasting your food, concentrating on one mouthful at a time, leaving food on your plate, exercising more and looking better and feeling better day after day. And what's more, you know that this is easy and enjoyable.

Looking in that mirror at the healthier, slimmer, shapely, more attractive you, that one-of-a-kind individual with an abundance of confidence and self-esteem, allows you to overcome all sorts of challenges in your life. The image in that mirror is real, your determination to achieve any goal is real, and your confidence is real. You are that image, see who you really are through that image, you know that this is easy and enjoyable, because you have already achieved it. You are looking at the results of your lifestyle change, and nothing can prevent you from bringing them to pass.

The Author:

Sarah Lamont has been a complementary therapist & healer for sixteen years, specialising in hypnotherapy. Having worked in the public sector for over twenty-three years and at a senior level for ten, Sarah finally decided that she wanted to help people on a one-to-one basis rather than serve the community impersonally.

'I have always found job satisfaction in helping other people rather than just going to work for the money. Working at a senior level in a large organisation in a very demanding and stressful job, finally made me realise that the skills I had as a healer, and the personal experience that I had of trying to attain a healthy work-life balance would be better served helping others find their balance'.

Under the banner of Satori Life and Health (www.satori-life-health.co.uk), Sarah's ethos is about providing services that are all about finding personal balance within our hectic lives. She believes that using a natural approach to better health, through working with the body and mind, supports our inherent ability to heal and is the best gift we can bestow on ourselves.

THE HELPFUL BRICK

AUTHOR: CHARLOTTE KNAGGS

Personalisation:

This metaphor is about literally building inner confidence and realising that you are better than you think you are. It can be used with clients who have low self-esteem or a self-critical inner dialogue. And it shows how, with a bit of research, you can find out extraordinary things about everyday objects!

Before you begin, establish a few positive qualities that your client believes they already have, and some they would like to develop. If they struggle to be positive about themselves, ask what complimentary words those who are closest to them would use to describe them, for example, their friends, colleagues, or family.

I wonder if you have ever thought about how ordinary things can be extraordinary when you look at them carefully. Some of those things we take for granted and hardly see, even though they are all around us, every day. Things that have been made by humans for almost ten thousand years, but that we don't even notice, because people have very fixed ideas about what is ordinary, what is nothing special at all, and what isn't, and sometimes those ideas are not the case at all.

We all know something about making these judgements from when we were children, from when we started to learn from others what to value and what not to value. When we started to form ideas about ourselves, for example, by comparing ourselves to others – and children can be both very harsh critics of each other and hard on themselves, but they are young, and they don't have all the information that we have when we grow up and mature into adults. When we realise that there are lots of different ways to be and that we all have different strengths and talents, experience and skills.

And the ordinary thing that I was thinking about was a brick. Just an ordinary brick. We use them in our homes, but we don't attach much importance or value to an individual brick. We even have sayings like 'thick as a brick', and this suggests that the brick is really nothing special at all, just a thick block, maybe a little rough, often rather plain.

And what if a brick was to compare itself to other materials, such as sophisticated Italian marble, smooth and pleasantly cool to the touch, or exotic Brazilian granite, flecked with mica that sparkles as it catches the light of the sun, or elegant Arabian sandstone, that can be carved into ornate pillars or statues? Then the humble brick might start to believe that it was a very inferior kind of material indeed.

But I can tell you that this is not the case at all. The very great city of Rome, the eternal city, once the capital of the world, was born a city of bricks. Each Roman brick was made from the local soil, a combination of clay mixed with water, sand, straw and finely ground volcanic dust and ash; ingredients that were carefully mixed and then pressed by hand into wooden moulds, and left to dry in the warm, bright sun, then, later, they would be hard fired by baking them in big ovens.

A brick is a thing made up of all the elements, and then baked into a material that is strong and versatile, beautiful, and warm. Bricks can be laid with the creativity of an artist, to form almost anything the imagination can conjure up, from plain, blind walls to gracefully curved arches and lofty vaults, from delicate latticework windows to roofs and smart herringbone floors.

There really is no more flexible and creative building material than the brick, an uncomplicated object that has unlimited potential. Bricks have been used to create magnificent buildings and structures, that are strong, enduring, and impressive. And every architect, engineer, and artisan knows that bricks get even better as they age, they are strong, sturdy, and reliable, and they retain heat and absorb humidity. They have proved themselves over and over again.

Bricks are one of the oldest building materials, and humans have been building with them from the earliest of times: from ancient Mayan temples and pyramids to the sumptuous, decorative brickwork of Persian cultures and Moorish Spain; from the tallest brick building in the world, St Martin's church in Bavaria, to the rows and rows of grand townhouses in our major cities; and the viaducts that span our green valleys, allowing puffing trains to transport their precious cargo. Even to this day, bricks are still regarded as one of the best building materials there is.

So, you can see, there is nothing inferior about the brick, not at all. This is just a silly old idea, an outdated and unfair idea, one that we can give no more thought or meaning to.

And now, as you consider how bricks are truly wonderful objects that have proven themselves so valuable, and useful, and reliable, you can become aware of how individual bricks are attached to one another with mortar, stacked up on top of each other, laid end to end, overlapped and layered, to create just the right building or structure to meet whatever the need is. A wall, a church, a house, or something else, the potential really is unlimited.

You could say that bricks are a bit like the things we build our life from: our individual experiences and the positive things we take from them; the pieces of knowledge we pick up; the skills we acquire; the lessons we learn; the good and kind qualities we nurture. They are all bricks that we mix and mould and fire ourselves, and then put into our storehouse of useful materials.

We can join all these bricks together, and arrange them however we like, as creatively as we choose to. Bringing together all our strengths, our abilities, and our skills, brick by brick, they make us who we are.

And I wonder, now, if you can see in your mind all your wonderful bricks, arranged carefully in a big, warm, dry storehouse? These versatile, efficient and practical bricks. Take a moment to look at those bricks now, notice each one and what it looks like. I wonder what colour they are, perhaps a warm orange, or a deep terracotta, or a dark brownish red. And now notice the texture, are they smooth, or rough, are the edges neat or uneven, how do they feel to the touch? And how do they smell? Is there a particular smell you associate with them?

As you continue to look at your bricks, you realise that each brick represents something, perhaps you are aware now that they have words moulded onto them, take a really close look at those words now. You just instinctively know what those words are and what they mean, there may be bricks with words like

[insert the positive qualities that your client thinks they already have, such as calm, focussed, organised, helpful, and competent.]

I wonder what else you have in that storehouse.

You realise that all these bricks represent a positive quality, skill, ability, piece of knowledge, or attribute, and there are lots and lots of them. All here in your storehouse, being kept safe, waiting to be used.

You also notice that the words on the bricks have been formed out of clay, and you just know somehow that it was you who made those words by hand, and attached them to the bricks, one by one.

Take a few moments now to have a really good look around, see how the bricks are arranged neatly in your storehouse, in just the way that makes the most sense to you.

And now, I'd like you to find all the bricks with the qualities and skills that you need for the future, they are all there, and you just somehow know which brick is which. Find the bricks that represent

[*insert the positive qualities your client would like to develop. Then pause, to allow them to identify the right bricks.*]

That's really good, and, once you are satisfied that you have found all the right bricks, I'd like you to imagine now that you are putting them together, in just the right order, and just the right way. Creatively, with no constraints, you may even find that some of the bricks are bigger than other bricks, or slightly different shades or colours, or textures. But you can find just the right shape and colour for the space, making building with your bricks even easier, and effortless.

That's right, and you can be sure that those bricks representing all your positive qualities will never run out, there is an unlimited supply of them in your storehouse, and you are adding more bricks all the time as you go through life. And you can also see that you can build a wonderful, creative representation of your capabilities at any time you like, allowing your powerful subconscious to put all those skills and attributes together in just the right way, to build that powerful story of what you can do, and how amazing you are.

The Author:

Charlotte Knaggs says of herself: I am a qualified hypnotherapist, reiki practitioner and shamanic healing practitioner based in Wakefield, West Yorkshire. Several things led me to want to train as a hypnotherapist. My first contact with hypnotherapy was around twenty years ago when I experienced a painful bereavement and then relocated to a new home two hundred and fifty miles away. I knew I needed to regain a positive mindset and improve my self-esteem and had a wonderful therapist who helped me a great deal. I have used the self-hypnosis techniques this therapist taught me at different points in my life – to manage anxiety, increase motivation and boost my self-belief.

More recently, while working as a senior manager in the Civil

Service, it hit me one day that I was on the brink of burnout. Some time out allowed me to reflect on my priorities, values and skills. I was already interested in providing therapeutic support through reiki and shamanic healing and I had wonderful memories of the hypnotherapist that helped me so much. As an English graduate, I have always had a passion for language and stories, so a seed was planted that has since flourished into a private practice. I love helping clients make the changes they want to using hypnotherapy techniques and happily work with a wide variety of issues. The most rewarding outcome, though, is working with a client's self-confidence and self-belief and seeing them let go of their limiting beliefs and self-doubt.

THREE KEYS
AUTHOR: ROSIE CATHRO

Personalisation:

Before beginning, you need to identify three things that your client *wants to feel, such as confident, calm, strong, etc. These are referred to in the script as A, B, and C; just swap them out where they are indicated. It's always best to use the client's own descriptors here, so either ask them to tell you three things that will help them or pick out relevant words from their conversation.*

You could start in the client's peaceful place and take a path or corridor from there to the country garden if you wish. If their peaceful place is already a garden, suggest they notice a small path they haven't seen before leading to a new part of it.

And you could make the coat their favourite colour, if you know it.

You find yourself on a winding path in a country garden, with a short hedge and a beautiful lawn on either side of the path. There are beautiful, curved flowerbeds too, following the course of the path.

There's a cool breeze, but you're wrapped up nice and warm, and you have a big, luxurious coat on, with a soft collar. In front of you, not too far in the distance, you see that your path is blocked by a big stone wall.

You wonder at first how you are going to get past this, but then you notice that the pathway leads you to a door. You continue walking along the path towards the big, wooden door which you see has beautiful patterns carved into it, and the words 'Your Future' on a bright and shining silver plaque.

You wonder again how you are going to open the door to get to the other side and continue to your future. You realise that you feel completely calm and confident that you will be able to do this, it's just a puzzle you need to solve, and you know you can do it.

You notice that there are three locks on the door, one labelled [A], the second labelled [B], and the third labelled [C].

In the coat you're wearing, the pockets are full of keys, and you realise these all represent different parts of you. Although you have doubted whether you have these qualities in the past, at this moment you realise you can reject all the negative beliefs you have previously held about yourself and you feel sure you can open the door.

You try each key in turn and the first lock that opens is the one labelled [A]. As the key opens the lock, you realise straight away that

[insert a description of what having more of that feeling would be like, such as 'you deserve to feel good about yourself.]

You decide that, once this door opens, this is definitely a key you will put back in your pocket and carry with you into your future.

You continue to try more keys. The next one that works is for the lock labelled [B]. You decide that once the door opens this is a key you will put back into your pocket too, to carry forward into your future as a reminder of

[insert an explanation of why this is important to the client, with examples of the changes they will be able to make in situations that have been difficult for them before.]

You find yourself with one more key to try and one lock to open, it's the lock labelled [C].

It's a shiny key, perhaps it's not been used as often as it should be, but it looks beautiful, and you pause to admire it for a moment. As you turn it, the lock springs open and the door to your future opens easily on its hinges. You realise that at this moment you can see a better future

[*insert a description of how, when and why the feelings will be useful in the future.*]

You feel a sense of pride and achievement rush through your body, it's such an amazing feeling.

You collect the keys you have used one by one, putting each of them back into your pocket. You are ready to step through the door and carry these keys with you into your future.

You know now that you can use these keys to help you unlock the door to any obstacle at any time.

These keys and attributes belong to you – you have earned them, and they are yours to use whenever you wish.

The Author:

Rosie Cathro is a professional Hypnotherapist and Coach. She says of herself:

I support women and mums to unravel the many 'shoulds' they have collected over time, so they can release the need for perfectionism and rediscover their identity. We work together to design a life that really works for them and that welcomes joy, balance, and ease. I'm based in West Yorkshire and work exclusively online, both 1:1 and via online courses.

My website is www.rosiecathrohypnotherapy.co.uk and you can find me on Instagram and Facebook by searching Rosie Cathro Hypnotherapy.

CHAPTER FOUR

CLEARING METAPHORS

In this chapter, you'll find clearing metaphors, which are designed to encourage the client to clear out and let go of underlying contributory factors such as past experiences which created their unhelpful thoughts, feelings, behaviour, or resistance. A kind of mental spring cleaning, if you wish (which, of course, would make a perfectly good clearing metaphor in its own right, at the right time of year.)

Most have themes of releasing burdens, making choices about what to keep and what to let go, and reimagining a future free from past problems. Sometimes authors suggest specific places for you to include the client's own experiences but, even if they don't, look for places you can do this to make them even more meaningful.

Clearing metaphors provide a good alternative to analytical techniques such as parts or regression where there is a reason not to confront these issues directly; for example, you have a limited number of sessions with the client and/or don't want to trigger conscious awareness of issues that they aren't yet ready to deal with.

Using clearing themes that are familiar to the client is the best way to go, for example, a fishing theme for someone who has that hobby. We don't have that one (maybe next time), but the process of sorting which kind of bait to use and which fish to keep or throw back suggests a host of possibilities.

THE LITTLE TOY CART
AUTHOR: SARAH LAMONT

Personalisation:

T his script includes the opportunity to refer to specific issues or circumstances that the client needs to release. So, before you start, *make sure you know:*

- *What is the issue, thought, or situation they want to clear?*
- *What will the change look like after it has taken place?*

The story taps into ideas about childhood and carefree days, with symbols of a toy cart, marbles, and a protective figure, so might be particularly useful for clients who had a secure upbringing.

You can, of course, transform the gate guardian into a specific person, if you know of someone who plays that role for the client, or a spiritual figure such as an angel, if that fits with their beliefs.

Now that you are feeling relaxed, it might be possible to allow yourself to switch off your thoughts, letting all your cares and worries just drift away. The outside world can fade into the background and any noises that you hear simply make you even more relaxed. The sound of my voice helps you relax even more.

Slowly take a deep breath in, then let it out as slowly as you can. A slow, steady, relaxing breath, feeling any remaining tension and anxiety melt away with that out-breath. You may even notice now how much more relaxed your body feels, feeling calm and contented, safe and secure.

I wonder if you can begin to imagine that you are walking down a country lane. The road is quiet and there is no sign of human life around you. It's a beautiful day and your favourite time of year, and it is the perfect temperature, you feel relaxed and at ease, as you walk along.

Ahead of you, you notice a gate that takes you off the lane. At the gate, you notice someone or something waiting for you. This could be a person from your past, present, or future, it could even be an animal, or something entirely different, but as you approach, they open the gate for you, closing it safely and securely behind you as you pass through.

As you greet one another you may even feel a wave of calm pass over you, giving you the sense that this is a safe haven, your safe haven, and that the company that you are in is like a guardian, someone with whom you can leave all your cares and worries.

They hand you what looks like a children's pull-along cart: notice the colour, does it mean anything to you? if you like, you can even bend down and inspect it closer.

[*Pause to allow the client to do this.*]

On the cart, you notice a box that is covered so that you can't see inside. Whilst this piques your interest, you know that you will find out soon enough what it contains and are happy not to investigate further for the moment.

Your companion points in the direction of a small path and you know without them saying anything that you would like to walk this path, so pulling the little cart behind you, you set off.

You can't help but observe how beautiful the day is as you walk along. You notice how quiet this place is, your own place where you can be peaceful and calm. The colours appear very vibrant, wonderful colours, you can even pause awhile to notice the delicate fragrances in the air, breathing in not only the scents, but a sense of peace which fills your lungs with every breath, leaving you feeling calm, you may even hear the calls of the birds or other wildlife around you.

As you continue walking along the path, you notice that you are feeling lighter and lighter, any negative thoughts or feelings you had seem to be lifting, like a weight is being lifted from your shoulders.

[*Pause to allow the client to experience this.*]

At the same time, you notice that the cart that you're pulling feels heavier and heavier, as though all your negativity is being transferred to the covered box in your cart, and as you walk further you continue to feel brighter, more relaxed, weightless even. Your sense of calm is effortless, it feels so natural.

Wow! Who would have thought you could experience such a sense of peace and tranquillity? Nothing matters, all that negativity has drifted into the box on the cart, it is almost as though the only thing that is stopping you from floating away is the weight of the cart behind you and your hand holding the handle.

I would like you, if you want to, to continue along this path until you either feel so light that you can barely keep your feet on the ground or until the weight of the cart is so heavy that you can no longer pull it any further. When that happens just say 'stop'.

[*Leave the client to follow the path, transferring the weight to the cart. If this seems to be taking a while, don't nag but encourage them by saying – you're feeling lighter and lighter and the cart is feeling heavier and heavier, just let me know when you want to stop by saying 'stop'. Once they say stop, continue.*]

Ahead of you, you can see a seat, so walk over and sit down for a rest. Just take a moment to feel this sense of peace, you may even notice how much calmer you feel, all the tension seems to have gone from your entire body, your head feels clear and totally free for the first time in so long, and your body is relaxed, your mind unwinding even more as you sit quietly and comfortably, and you can finally let go of any remaining unwanted, unnecessary negative thoughts and feelings. That's it, let it all go, what a welcome relief.

Now turn your attention to the cart and open the box. Inside you notice lots and lots of marbles, no wonder the cart was so heavy. The box is so full, and on the very top of the marbles is a very special magnifying glass. Pick up the magnifying glass and choose one of the marbles. Take your time and look closely into the marble, can you see the writing inside? If you can't, adjust the distance of the marble with the magnifying glass, can you see it now? It says:

[*insert whatever the issue or situation is that they are feeling negative about.*]

Just think, each marble contains one of the things that held you back,

[*insert examples of things they felt negative about or negative thoughts they have experienced*]

and all these thoughts and feelings have now transferred from you to the marbles in your cart. No wonder you feel so much lighter, so much calmer, and so very, very relaxed.

As you sit there now, notice you no longer feel

[*insert their past responses to the situation they want to release, and how that negativity presented.*]

It's all gone. No wonder you feel so good.

It feels right to now move back along the path that you have walked, but before you do, you turn the cart around and look at the back of the cart. Can you see there is a marble-sized cork at the bottom of the box? Even if you can't, that's not a problem, you can just imagine yourself pulling the cork out, that's great. You can now start to walk back to the gate that you came through.

As you walk along the path, you notice that the marbles are falling out of the box and rolling away. You feel the cart becoming lighter as the weight of these marbles is released from the box, releasing you to experience even more delightful feelings of inner calm and confidence. No longer pulling along all those concerns, all that negativity in your day-to-day life, but experiencing a feeling of being at ease with yourself. And when you're at ease with yourself, how much more natural it seems to feel at ease with the world around you. As you continue to walk along the path, you can allow your imagination free rein to run through all the occasions in your life which you will experience from now on with a calm sense of self, with more courage and with more ease and confidence than you ever had before, more than you ever thought possible.

[*Future pacing – insert some examples of the client coping positively with situations that would have been problematic in the past.*]

It seems so natural, how simple this was. To go for a walk and to shed all those negative thoughts or feelings and replace them with a sense of calm, serenity, and composure, which will allow you to go through your daily life with ease and peace. How simple was this, how easy it has been.

As you reach the gate your companion is there waiting for you, and you hand over the empty cart to them. You know that if your negative thoughts or feelings ever get on top of you again in the future, you can return to this wonderful place, and your companion will be waiting for you at the gate with your negativity cart. You now know how easy it is to shed those thoughts and concerns, how much better you feel after offloading the weight, to leave you feeling calm and positive. You walk through the gate and your companion closes it securely behind you.

As you begin to reorient yourself back to the here and now, you can enjoy this wonderful sense of feeling lighter and uplifted, with a wonderful sense of ease and calm confidence in your mind, body, and spirit that will stay with you in the coming hours, days, weeks, and months. And you return to full awareness of how calm, positive, and revitalised you truly feel.

The Author:

Sarah Lamont has been a complementary therapist & healer for sixteen years, specialising in hypnotherapy. Having worked in the public sector for over twenty-three years and at a senior level for ten, Sarah finally decided that she wanted to help people on a one-to-one basis rather than serve the community impersonally.

'I have always found job satisfaction in helping other people rather than just going to work for the money. Working at a senior level in a large organisation in a very demanding and stressful job, finally made me realise that the skills I had as a healer, and the personal experience that I had of trying to attain a healthy work-life balance would be better served helping others find their balance'.

Under the banner of Satori Life and Health (www.satori-life-health.co.uk), Sarah's ethos is about providing services that are all about finding personal balance within our hectic lives. She believes that using a natural approach to better health, through working with the body and mind, supports our inherent ability to heal and is the best gift we can bestow on ourselves.

THE PEBBLE TOWERS
AUTHOR: VANESSA PLACE

Personalisation:

T his can be tied in with the client's peaceful place if that's a beach, or with a specific beach if you know of one that the client likes visiting.

If the client prefers the countryside or a garden, you can adapt the opening paragraphs to have them walk there until they come upon a beach, or an open space of natural pebbles near a stream.

If you change the setting, don't forget to throw the pebbles 'as far as you can' rather than 'out to sea', to omit mention of waves lapping and receding, to change the beach hut to something more suitable for the environment, (perhaps replacing it with a shed or cave) and to breathe in the fresh air rather than the fresh sea air.

Before you begin you will need to establish:

- *The client's goals and the resources they need to achieve them, such as confidence, motivation etc.]*
- *Examples of thoughts, feelings or behaviours the client wants to leave behind, such as skin picking, anxiety, smoking, and overeating.*

This metaphor combines the clearing process with a powerful example of standing strong against future adversity, so might be particularly useful for clients who are in an ongoing or recurring stressful situation.

As you continue relaxing, deeper and deeper now, I'd like you to imagine that you are walking along a beautiful sandy beach. You can be barefoot or have something on your feet – I wonder which you prefer? Overhead, the sky is blue, with just the occasional white fluffy cloud drifting by. The warm sun feels so good on your skin. And as you walk along your breathing is calm and steady, just enjoy breathing in the fresh sea air, that's right – so fresh, so pure.

Any old stress or tension is easily removed now, with each and every breath out. That's right – just breathe out any old stress or tension. That's good. That's right. It's a beautiful day, and you're enjoying walking along the beach.

Keep walking for a while, just walking along. Perhaps you notice the soft sand beneath your feet, or perhaps the sound of the gulls calling to each other, just keep walking for a while longer, that's right, walking on, until you reach an area at the end of the beach, a place where the sand fades, and in its place are thousands of pebbles, pebbles of all shapes and sizes, pebbles for as far as the eye can see.

Amongst all these pebbles, people who passed this way before you have created hundreds of pebble towers. In fact, there are towers of pebbles stretching far into the distance. These towers stretch out before you now, some small, others quite tall. Some are balanced perfectly, some look a bit haphazard, and others have fallen down. An amazing sight!

[*Pause to allow the client time to imagine this.*]

All the towers are unique in their own special way. Mesmerised, you gaze out across the view, intrigued by all the different pebble towers. And then, on impulse – you decide to create one too!

So, carefully look around now and choose your pebbles.

Pebbles which will create your perfect tower. Pebbles the right size, shape and colour to work together in harmony, creating that perfect balance. Pebbles that will support each other, creating a strong tower.

[*Pause.*]

Notice the feel of each pebble as you pick it up, cool and smooth perhaps, or rough and uneven. Wet, damp, or perhaps perfectly dry. Maybe even a little sandy, gritty between your fingertips. Some are a heavy weight in your hand, and others are hardly noticeable.

And, as you choose your pebbles, make sure to include plenty representing

[*include examples of the client's chosen resources.*]

Because these are the qualities you want and deserve to have. And you will, once they are in your tower. That's great work.

Now, sometimes you find that unwanted pebbles make it into a collection, perhaps without a person really noticing they were there. These are the pebbles which could cause a tower to wobble, or even fall! So, any unhelpful pebbles in your collection need discarding before you build your tower.

Allow your mind to check now for any unsuitable pebbles which you might already have but no longer want in your life, pebbles which might represent

[*include examples of thoughts, behaviour or feelings that the client wants to release.*]

And when you find a pebble representing those unwanted habits, grasp it tightly in your hand, reach back your arm, and fling it far out to sea. That's right. Any unsuitable pebbles in your collection, the ones you don't want in your tower, the ones that don't belong there, find them now and launch them right out to sea, so they're out of sight, and out of mind – allowing the waves to take them away, gone for good.

Good work, that's right. You easily know which pebbles are just right, the ones you need to keep because they represent all the strengths you already have, as well as all your new desired strengths and behaviours. Keep only the best pebbles now and replace any of the ones you discarded with more suitable, helpful new ones.

Take as long as you need, carefully checking through your collection. Throw away those unhelpful ones, the ones that you no longer want or need. And give me a nod when you've done that.

[*Wait for the nod.*]

You now have only pebbles that will balance together perfectly. Pebbles that will allow you to build your wonderful tower – strong, confident, positive, amazing. In fact, everything you would like it to be. That's right. And when you have gathered all the pebbles that you need, and cast away those which are wobbly, uneven, or just don't feel right, then make your way over to a little clearing by the water's edge and begin building your tower. Good, that's right. Working steadily now, you make careful and positive choices, using only the best pebbles, adding more if necessary, removing or swapping some as needed. And, in doing so, create your perfect tower.

That's right, that's good. And since each pebble represents different parts of you, your thoughts, feelings, memories, and behaviours too, you know how important it is to choose each pebble with care, creating your perfect tower steadily, and carefully. Take your time. A tower of pebbles near the water's edge. Perfectly balanced. Build until you are happy with the pebbles you have included, take your time, and when it is finished, give me a little nod.

[*Wait for the nod.*]

A strong tower has emerged. You've worked hard, so now is the time to sit and rest for a while, enjoying the peace, enjoying the calm, enjoying your achievement, as you listen to the waves gently lapping up and receding, lapping up and receding. Your breathing is slow and steady now, each breath in fills you with a wonderful feeling of calm, of positivity, and each breath out removes any remaining worry or stress. That's right, just enjoy this feeling of being so calm, so relaxed. That's good.

Now, after a while, you decide it's time to move on, but as you start to walk back the way you came the sky begins to darken – there's a storm brewing in the distance, and dark clouds are heading your way.

Looking around, you notice an empty beach hut. Go over there and give the door a push, step inside to shelter until the storm passes. That's right, make yourself comfortable in there. Safe from the storm outside. Rest a little longer, safe in the beach hut, protected from the wind, protected from the rain.

After a while, the storm passes, as all storms do, and you emerge from your shelter. Looking up, you see the sky is blue again, and the warm sun feels so good on your skin. The sun's warming rays fill you now with new energy, a new sense of wellbeing. Just enjoy that pleasant feeling, absorb it all, and keep it within you. That's good. That's right.

You feel curious to see how your tower has coped in the storm, so go back to have a look. And there it is, standing firm, looking good! Only a couple of pebbles have moved a little out of place. See yourself smiling now as you quickly readjust and repair your tower – finding this so easy to do! Still smiling, you notice a new confidence within you, a new confidence and an ability to calmly deal with any storms which come your way from now on. A new confidence and motivation within you now to move forward with all these positive new changes.

The changes you desired are now in place within your unconscious mind. They grow in strength over the days to come, giving you the power to achieve whatever you wish to achieve. Because this is your wish. Go on with the rest of your day now. Feeling energised. Those old thoughts and feelings no longer weigh you down or bother you in any way now, you feel lighter, free and ready. There is a new confidence within you. Because now you know how to re-adjust, re-balance your tower any time you need to. Well done.

The Author:

Vanessa Place qualified as a hypnotherapist in 2018 following her training in York with YHT. Her practice – www.peacefulplacehypnotherapy.com – is situated in beautiful North Yorkshire, where her therapy room looks out over the open countryside.

Before becoming a hypnotherapist, Vanessa was a nurse for thirty-five years, caring for both adults and children during her career, which included time working at Great Ormond Street Hospital in London.

Vanessa enjoys spending time with her family and walking in the countryside with Millie the family dog. She also has a love of Ibiza, visiting the island a few times each year to walk, party and watch the sunsets. It was, however, a beach in Tenerife which was the inspiration for 'The Pebble Tower'. Vanessa came across the pebble beach by chance while out walking, and of course, stopped to build one of her own. Vanessa's clients particularly like this metaphor, and she hopes you and your clients will do too.

WEEDS

AUTHOR: DEBBIE WALLER

Personalisation:

You have probably told clients many times that even feelings which seem negative or overwhelming, are, at a deeper level, protective. Anxiety, for example, is there to make us careful, to be ready for danger in places where it might suddenly jump out at us. It's only when feelings like this are not in proportion to the amount of risk we're facing that they feel like a liability instead of an asset.

This metaphor makes the point that, in the right place, all our feelings are valuable and useful. We don't need to be rid of them, only to encourage them to be what they were designed to be.

You can help client identification with the metaphor by giving the gardener a few characteristics they share, and by making their favourite plants prominent in the story. Make sure they aren't phobic about worms, bugs, or butterflies before mentioning these specifically!

There was once a gardener who was very proud of the garden he tended. He was out there every day, come rain or shine, mowing the grass, trimming and tying back the plants, and cutting flowers to take indoors.

The gardener worked hard in the garden, but he also took the time to enjoy it. Some days he would just sit out there and soak up the sights and smells, relaxing and feeling so good, surrounded by all his favourite plants and trees. There were always a few weeds around, of course, but he didn't really mind. 'After all,' he told himself, 'Weeds are just wildflowers, growing where they choose instead of where I decide to put them'.

And to be honest, a few weeds did the garden good. Where the soil didn't get much rain or sun, the more cultivated flowers wouldn't grow, but the weeds added a welcome bit of colour. The kind of weeds that grew told him about what nutrients the soil had or needed, and they attracted useful creatures – insects to pollinate and to feed on bugs that ate the leaves, worms to break down and feed the soil, and beautiful butterflies he could enjoy watching.

And some of the weeds were pretty, or even useful, so the gardener could enjoy a lovely dandelion tea as he relaxed in the garden or add chickweed and mallow to a salad at teatime.

Over time, though, the weeds began to grow stronger and stronger. They spread much faster than the cultivated flowers that the gardener wanted to grow, and they started to take over the garden. Where a few of them had been useful, a lot became overwhelming.

At first, the gardener didn't really notice. The number of weeds increased so slowly that it wasn't obvious at first just how much of a problem it was becoming. But, after a while, it became obvious that the beautiful plants he had loved to tend

[use the client's favourite plants if you know them]

were no longer thriving. They were being crowded out and starved of light, water, and food. Far from being useful, the weeds had become a big problem.

The gardener redoubled his efforts to keep the weeds at bay. He was out in the garden morning noon and night, hoeing and pulling out every single one, determined to get rid of them no matter what. heaping them all into the recycling bin or chopping, shredding and burning as many as he could. Sometimes, he didn't get to bed till really late and he no longer enjoyed his garden. It wasn't fun at all, it wasn't satisfying. It was just constant, back-breaking, exhausting work. He never got to sit out and appreciate the results of his labours because there were always weeds crushing and overpowering the plants he wanted to grow. In fact, sometimes it seemed that the harder he fought the weeds, the faster they grew until, eventually, he was too tired to even try. He saw the weeds as his enemy, and he knew they were winning.

One day, the gardener decided to try a new approach. Instead of pulling out the weeds and burning them, or throwing them away, he cleared an area of the garden to create a compost heap. And, right at the back of the garden, he chose an area to be a wildflower border.

He took the prettiest, most useful, and rarest of the weeds and transplanted them to the new wildflower area. He let them grow just as they wished, so now they had an appropriate place of their own, where they couldn't push out the other flowers. They grew, well, like wildflowers and once again they attracted bees, butterflies and other useful insects into the garden to help pollinate the cultivated flowers. So, in the right place, those weeds became useful again.

The rest, he pulled out and tumbled together on the compost heap where they gradually began to break down into a nutritious mulch that could be used to feed the cultivated plants. So, even the unwanted weeds were transformed into something that helped to make the garden healthier and better.

From that moment on, the gardener stopped trying to get rid of the weeds, he simply kept them in their own special place, where they benefited the rest of the garden without taking over. They were useful again, feeding the other plants, improving the soil, and attracting wildlife that helped the garden to grow.

And the gardener could enjoy his garden again, especially that dandelion tea when he sat down to rest.

The Author:

Debbie Waller is a hypnotherapist in Normanton, West Yorkshire. She is also a hypnotherapy supervisor and Director/Head Tutor of Yorkshire Hypnotherapy Training. She is the author of 'Their Worlds, Your Words', and 'The Hypnotherapist's Companion', a contributor to the 'Hypnotherapy Handbook' and past editor of the 'Hypnotherapy Journal'. And of course, contributing editor of this book of metaphors.

THE WORRY RUCKSACK

AUTHOR: STEVE LOVATT

Personalisation:

T he following is a framework to be used for clients who tend to let their early life events affect them. In particular, the author says it has proven to be beneficial for clients who present with low mood and low self-esteem, but for no single event or reason. The script uses a series of metaphors around painful memories and utilises colours to signify value and beauty. Caution should be used before using this script for any severe trauma-related memories, as it has limited ability to allow full reprocessing.

Like the Pebble Tower, it uses the idea of stones to represent the emotional burdens the client has been carrying but, as you'll see, it's a completely different approach. Artistic clients, or those who rely on intuition, might enjoy the creativity of tower-building, whereas those who prefer structure, feeling in control and logic are likely to favour the more analytical sorting process offered here.

This could be personalised by making the footpath one that the client knows, perhaps where they walk their dog. Or by tying it into a holiday where they went walking, hiking or even mountaineering if this is something they enjoy.

. . .

As you relax, you begin to notice your breath. Without holding or controlling your breath, just let it happen, calmly, naturally, and relaxingly. Noticing how as you inhale the belly rises, and as you exhale the belly falls. How when inhaling the navel or belly button moves away from the spine and exhaling the navel or belly button drifts towards the spine, lifting and drifting – naturally, calmly, safely. Drifting gently into a deep relaxation, drifting deeper and deeper into a deep, calm, safe, relaxation.

[*Further hypnotic deepeners can be used here if you are working with trance.*]

As you relax, deeply, deeper and deeper, allow your imagination to open, like the pages of a photo album. Crisp, clear, vivid images, in sharp focus.

All you need to do is listen to the sound of my voice, knowing that you are in the right place, at the right time, with nowhere else to go, nothing else to do. Just relax and imagine vivid images or paintings. And, if you find it difficult to imagine images, then follow my narration by adding details in your mind in your own way.

Imagine that you are walking on a footpath on a perfect summer's day, not too hot and not too cold, under a cloudless blue sky. What colour blue is your perfect sky?

Notice a bright yellow/orange sun suspended in the sky, just floating, feeling the warmth against your face and skin, feeling completely safe and relaxed.

As you walk, you begin to notice how the weight is transferred from each foot to the other, one by one, one by one. Feeling the support of the ground, the earth beneath your feet. Feeling safe, grounded, relaxed, content, and free.

As you walk, feeling relaxed, you notice nature all around you, the plants, trees, and grasses. You notice evidence of nature all around you. You also become aware of thoughts and memories which have been weighing on your mind.

You now notice that you have a rucksack on your back. It feels heavy. Why does it feel so heavy? Why have you been carrying this rucksack for so long?

Find a suitable place, and take a seat on the ground, still feeling safe and grounded. Take the rucksack from your back and place it in front of you. Open the rucksack, and notice it is filled with rocks of all types, shapes, and colours. Place your hand in the rucksack and take out a particularly sharp, heavy rock.

Hold it in your hand, and notice its shape, texture, the sharp edges, the heavy weight, the colour. Is this something you feel you wish to keep, or is it just a weight that does not serve you, something you no longer want or need?

The choice is yours, it's up to you. If you feel this rock no longer serves any useful purpose, if indeed it ever did, place it on the ground to the side of you.

Now, take another rock from the rucksack, maybe this is a rock you feel you have been carrying for so long, longer than you really felt you had to. Notice the texture, colour, shape and weight of that one. Maybe it's smoother, but still heavy, maybe it's sharp and painful to hold, maybe it's just grey and uninteresting, offering no enjoyment or stimulation.

Perhaps you can remember when you first acquired this rock, maybe you have no idea when you first started carrying it. Maybe it has a purpose and connection, or maybe you wonder why you have carried it for so long? You can now make a choice with this rock, and if you decide you no longer want or need it you can place it beside the other rock on the ground.

Now spend a few minutes taking each of the heavy rocks out, one by one, one by one, one by one. Noticing how each rock feels, and how heavy it is. How sharp or rough it feels. What colour it is and whether you want or need it.

You can decide for each rock whether to place it in a pile of value, to keep and cherish, or to place it on the ground with the others that no longer serve you, the ones you no longer what or need.

Take your time, one rock at a time, and I'll stay quiet in the background for a few minutes to allow you to carefully remove each heavy rock.

[Pause for 1-2 minutes, whilst the client works their way through the rucksack, occasionally offering cues and support. If there are specific memories to be dealt with you can introduce specific rocks for these as suggestions. You could also ask the client to give you a nod when they've finished so you know you can go on.]

Please nod when you have taken all the heavy rocks from your rucksack

[Wait for the nod.]

Well done, you have done such an amazing job of considering, and sorting, all those rocks.

Now, with all the heavy rocks removed from the rucksack, you can become aware of smaller rocks that have maybe fallen to the bottom of the rucksack. Small, smooth, light rocks and stones. You take one of these from the bottom of the rucksack and place it in your hand, noticing how light it is, how smooth it is, noticing the delicate shape, the colour. Such a beautiful stone, such a colourful stone, a gemstone perhaps, your gemstone. Maybe you are wondering how you could have forgotten ever collecting this stone, maybe it was long, long ago.

As you look and marvel at this gemstone, you realise that this is the stone which brings joy, happiness, lightness and beauty, love. Place this stone in another small pile next to you.

Now take out another small, perfect stone from the rucksack and marvel at its qualities, the colour, shape, texture, and how light it feels. Marvel at this valuable stone, maybe forgotten for so long, or maybe recently collected on this journey we call life. Celebrate its value to you, and place this along with the other gemstone at your feet.

I will again be silent for a few minutes as you discover, or maybe rediscover, all the gemstones in your rucksack. One by one, one by one, one by one. That's right, noticing their individual beauty, colour, texture, and weight. Maybe some are red, orange, yellow, green, blue, indigo, or violet.

[Include the client's favourite colour or the name of their favourite crystal, if you know it.]

Each one is a thing of beauty, precious and valuable. Each one is placed with the other gemstones on the ground.

[*Pause to allow the client to discover each gemstone.*]

And when you are ready, please nod when you have found all the gemstones in your rucksack.

[*Wait for the nod.*]

Well done, such an impressive collection of beautiful, colourful, valuable stones. Now, take each of these valuable stones in turn and place them carefully, safely back in the rucksack.

Now, look at the pile of stones which you hadn't decided to keep or discard, are there ANY of these which serve you or that you would like to keep?

Take your time. You can place one or more of these back in your rucksack if you want to, but you don't have to keep any. It's up to you.

Now, look at the pile of heavy, sharp, unattractive stones, the ones you no longer want or need, that do not serve you. As you look at this pile of stones, you notice they are slowly sinking, drifting into the ground, slowly being absorbed by the earth, this mother earth.

As you watch, it's almost as if time is speeding up as you witness these stones getting smaller and smaller, smaller and smaller, until they are tiny, tiny, tiny. Until, they are gone, gone, gone.

Place the rucksack back on your shoulders and notice how light it feels. How a great weight, a burden, has been lifted from your shoulders. A weight off your mind.

Notice how easy it is to continue your walk, feeling confident and happy, observing the wonders of nature, feeling the warmth of the sun, on this perfect day.

Allow a feeling of confidence, freedom and love to fill every bone, muscle, tendon, ligament, organ, every cell of your body, feeling a release from the weight of carrying anything that you no longer wanted or needed, that did not serve you.

The Author:

Steve Lovatt is a holistic hypnotherapist, Soma breath coach, Theta healer, dream yoga facilitator, mindfulness practitioner, mindful meditation practitioner, and sound therapist. Working from his private practice at the edge of the Yorkshire Dales, he has a particular interest in anxiety and trauma release, using a tapestry of modalities to guide through healing pathways, using a journey of discovery within the subconscious mind. He also is a lecturer for a national training provider, training therapists in the areas of anxiety release, trauma, PTSD, and CPTSD. He works with several corporate clients, using his extensive corporate experience to assist them in their staff wellbeing programmes. Steve's website can be found at www.yourtimewellness.uk.

CHAPTER FIVE

FAIRY TALES AND THE WISDOM
OF OLD WIVES

In this chapter, you'll find metaphors that are inspired by familiar stories and sayings, though they often have a bit of a twist or an unusual point of view to make more impact therapeutically.

They appeal to the child within us and are suitable for most clients.

Hopefully, they will also give you the inspiration to take idioms and sayings that the client uses and create healing stories of your own.

CINDERELLA

AUTHOR: DEBBIE WALLER

Personalisation:

J ust to put this in perspective, Marian Roalfe Cox[1] identified three
hundred and forty-five variants of the Cinderella story, including
some with a masculine protagonist. But that was in 1892, and the
number must have grown considerably since. And, since we can never
have too much of a good thing, here's one more.

*I originally wrote this for a client with 'empty nest syndrome' – all
the kids had grown up and gone, and she needed the confidence to go back
to being herself instead of as 'Mum' and start developing her career. It's
also worked well for me as a metaphor for feeling undervalued and
finding lost confidence in other situations. It can, of course, also be
adapted as a reminder to clients who think you're going to do all the
work, the message being that therapy, like magic, only helps if the client
does their bit.*

Or perhaps I just like the idea of myself as a Fairy Godmother.

What you were telling me about your situation made me think of a
story I was reading to my children recently.

It's the story of Cinderella who, as you probably know, found herself living as a servant in what should have been her own home, and looking after people who didn't seem to value what she did at all. It didn't matter how hard she worked, how good she was at what she did, or how cheerful and supportive she tried to be. They simply took it for granted and expected more. And the only tasks they did notice were the ones she didn't have time to do.

Cinderella didn't complain, of course, she just carried on, putting everyone else's needs ahead of her own, and doing her best at whatever tasks she was given whether she was appreciated or not. But she got out of the way of going out into the world. She lost touch with the friends she'd had in happier days and found herself getting used to her own company.

One day, an invitation came to go to a ball at the Palace. The prince was looking for a wife and had decided that he would interview every unmarried lady in the kingdom for the job by getting them all in the same place at the same time. It was a very practical solution, even if not a very romantic one.

Cinderella was really excited. Although it seemed unlikely the prince would choose her, if she wasn't there, a small chance became no chance at all. And to Cinderella, being chosen wasn't really the point. This was her big chance to get out of the rut she was in, to move into a larger world again, to meet new people, and to do new things.

But, of course, her sisters didn't want her to go. They didn't like washing up or cleaning, and they were happier with her in the house doing everything for them. Perhaps they even had a sense that Cinderella was the heroine of her own story, and unusual coincidences were likely to happen. But, faced with their disapproval, Cinderella said to herself, 'Maybe it's best just to stay at home then; after all, I haven't got a dress, and I'm not used to going to parties anymore. I'll probably be happier here by myself, reading a book'.

Now, in the story I read to my children, Cinderella was lucky enough to have a Fairy Godmother and she came along and solved

Cinders' problems for her so that she could live happily ever after. Or at least, that's the way most people tell the tale.

But, as I was reading that story, it occurred to me that, if I was Cinderella, I'd want my Fairy Godmother to have a much better magic wand.

What I'd really want is to be picked up from that lonely fireplace and zapped straight into the prince's arms – whirling elegantly in my beautiful dress.

Or (given that my dancing would be unlikely to impress) straight into the proposal scene. Or better still, the wedding.

No complications.

No mice, no pumpkin, no curfew.

No obscure search that might put the wrong girl with the right-sized feet in my place by his side.

But it isn't like that at all, is it? It's, 'Here's the dress, here's the coach. Now go get him. But you must do it before 12 o'clock.'

Imagine how it must have felt.

You arrive late and quite alone; the Fairy Godmother has left you to it. The palace gardens are quiet, but you can hear music and voices coming from inside.

You step out of the carriage and find your way to the ballroom.

Everyone stops, stares, and the whispers start.

The prince is intrigued, he comes forward and speaks to you.

Was it really all done by magic? No.

Despite the Rolls Royce coach and free designer clothes, the courage to open the ballroom door and walk into that room came from inside Cinderella herself. She found it left over from a time when she had been free to go to parties, to have friends, and to be happy, to be her real self.

And if she hadn't done that then she'd have spent her evening sitting alone in the pumpkin coach on the palace drive, dreaming about what might have been. The dress, the mice and all the rest of it would have been no good to her at all.

If you think about it, the magic wand didn't solve Cinders'

problems. It simply gave her a way to find the answers inside herself – just as this session does for you.

The Author:

Debbie Waller is a hypnotherapist in Normanton, West Yorkshire. She is also a hypnotherapy supervisor and Director/Head Tutor of Yorkshire Hypnotherapy Training. She is the author of 'Their Worlds, Your Words', and 'The Hypnotherapist's Companion', a contributor to the 'Hypnotherapy Handbook' and past editor of the 'Hypnotherapy Journal'. And of course, contributing editor of this book of metaphors.

COUNTING SHEEP

AUTHOR: KATHLEEN ROBERTS

Personalisation:

We all know that counting sheep is supposed to help us get to sleep and this story builds on that to help clients with insomnia, although it would be great for worrying as well, since it includes elements of letting go and just being in the moment. Just change the references at the end so instead of talking about 'when you lie in bed' it refers to 'when you start to worry'. Bear in mind that some places where clients experience anxiety or worrying may not be safe environments to close their eyes, so you can simply suggest that they 'remember the shepherd and sheep in whatever way is safe and comfortable' instead.

It could be personalised by setting it in their preferred peaceful place, if that's a suitable country scene, or perhaps by referring to a holiday or walk they had with their family, if you know of one.

Really take your time reading this, leaving long pauses between each phrase so the client has time to imagine the things you are talking about, and the repetition of language helps them to relax.

. . .

While you are in this deep state of relaxation, I'd like you to think about those times when you've been trying to sleep, and you might have tried the old trick of counting sheep.

I'd like you to imagine them now, trotting across a field in groups. A few of them jumping over a low dry-stone wall, or going through an open farm gate, or just wandering about on the grass, as you try to count them. Trying to get them into some kind of order, trying to count them one at a time, under the blue summer sky, on the hillside, with a river far below you in the bottom of the dale, water shining in the valley, and birds singing in the distance.

But instead of behaving themselves and staying quiet and still in the field, letting you count them in order, or proceeding one at a time through the gate, or climbing carefully and slowly onto the wall each, in turn, they mill about and crowd together.

They charge in different directions, they rush at the wall and scramble headlong over it, they jostle through the gate in panic.

And you know that the more you try to control those sheep, the more you try to count how many there are, the less they do what you want them to, the less orderly they are, the less you can control them, under the blue summer sky, on the hillside, with the river far below you in the bottom of the dale, water shining in the valley, and birds singing in the distance.

Because those sheep are just sheep, and sheep need a shepherd, and a sheepdog to organise them, to have some authority over them, to make them into an orderly flock. To calm them down and take control, to make them feel relaxed and safe, so that they can slow down, placidly and calmly, Into an orderly flock.

And now you can see the sheepdog enter the field, and the shepherd is leaning over the wall, and he is calling to his dog, very quietly. Giving orders to the dog, very calmly, with perfect assurance.

"Come by, come by."

You notice then, that straight away, the sheep become still, and calm.

Because they know the dog, because they trust the shepherd, because they can now relax.

They have confidence in the shepherd, they can feel safe now that they've seen the dog, and they know that now someone is in control.

Now there is order. Now there is safety. Now everything is as it should be.

Nothing is left to chance.

Everything is in its right place.

Now they can relax and feel that sense of relaxation, that feeling of comfort, surround them. Under the blue summer sky, on the hillside, with the river far below you at the bottom of the dale, water shining in the valley, and birds singing in the distance.

And now you notice that those sheep are waiting patiently, lining up, a leader at the front, waiting for the shepherd to walk along the side of the field and open the gate at the end of it. Just wide enough, just open enough, for a single sheep to pass through it easily.

But only one at a time.

And all the sheep, calm now, completely relaxed, all in a group, amble towards the gate.

Contentedly, thinning out, forming into single file, watched by the shepherd, leaning over the wall, nodding to his dog.

Both working as a team, they are organised, orderly, managing the sheep, who are calm and relaxed, and contented.

The shepherd himself is calm and relaxed, confident.

He has done this a thousand times before.

He will do it a thousand times again. Under the blue summer sky, on the hillside, with the river far below you at the bottom of the dale, water shining in the valley, and birds singing in the distance.

The first sheep ambles towards the gate, towards the gap, and through the open gate, the others, in formation, close behind.

And now you can count those sheep very easily, along with the shepherd, as those sheep amble through the gate, one at a time, calm and relaxed.

Counting those sheep, along with the shepherd, his lips moving very slightly, as he counts, his eyes resting on the sheep as they amble slowly through the open gateway.

Unconcerned, relaxed, calm.

The blue sky above you, warm in the sun, clouds scudding over the hills, and birdsong coming from the dale below, where the silver river flows.

Not only can you count the sheep now, one at a time, keeping track of them all, but you can check each one, make sure it is healthy, make sure it is fine, and make sure that all is as it should be.

You allow yourself to notice everything. You are watchful and careful, mindful of all the things you need to know. The sheep are content, each one is healthy, the grass in the field is rich and plentiful, and the dry-stone walls of the field are in good repair. There are no gaps in any of them, no missing stones, no holes where a sheep could get through. The stile over the wall is well-maintained, the gate has a secure latch, it closes on a spring so that it can't be left open by accident.

The dog is well-trained, and good at his job, he can be relied upon to control the sheep calmly, and with authority, to obey every order instantly.

And I'd just like you to take a minute to enjoy that feeling of being able to relinquish control to the shepherd. Of feeling confident that things are in order, that everything is as it should be, that feeling of relaxation and calm.

Just enjoy it for a moment, under the blue sky, looking down into the dale, listening to the birdsong, conscious of the sun and its warmth, of the river flowing placidly below.

Nothing to worry about, nothing to even think about. Just the enjoyment of the blue summer sky,

And the birds singing in the distance.

[*Leave a pause.*]

And before you allow yourself to drift back up into conscious wakefulness and awareness, I'd like you to think about those feelings, and how good they feel to you. How you can make them happen when you need to, every day.

I'd like you to think about how you can make them part of your everyday life, that feeling of calmness, of being in control, and being able to let go of responsibility when you wish to. The feeling that everything is in order and as it should be.

[*Leave a pause.*]

Now I'd like you to take a last look at the sheep, grazing now in the adjoining field. The shepherd is striding off down the hill, his dog is at his side. He turns at the field gate and gives you a wave. And you know that you can go back to that place. You know the way there so well, it's always there for you.

And when you lie in bed at night, ready to revisit this place, relinquishing the part of the day that your conscious mind inhabits, you close your eyes and again you see the sheep in the field. You know that at any moment you will see the shepherd, and you know that he will take charge. And that nothing needs attention, because it's in his capable hands.

Under the blue summer sky, on the hillside, with the river far below you at the bottom of the dale, water shining in the valley, and birds singing in the distance.

And you will be able to drift off to the sound of birdsong, letting go and leaving things to the shepherd, drifting into a deep and nourishing sleep.

But now, I'd like you to begin to leave that place, leaving everything in order, safe and secure, orderly, and calm.

Just for now.

The Author:

Kathleen Roberts is a former journalist, lecturer and local authority officer. She trained as a hypnotherapist with Yorkshire Hypnotherapy Training and is now one of their independent assessors. She also works as an educational consultant and is one of a panel of expert assessors for the EU's Erasmus+ scheme.

ELYSIAN FIELDS

AUTHOR: BRIAN TURNER

Personalisation:

T his is to help people process grief, which you will come across in many forms within a practice.

The Elysian fields are a place in Greek Mythology where those favoured by the gods went to spend the rest of their existence. Essentially, it's their version of Heaven. There is no pain or suffering, only happiness and joy, and this makes it ideal for working with grief.

However, you do not have to refer to it by its Greek name, and to be fair I seldom do. You need not give it a spiritual context unless you want to and feel that the client will respond. It can simply be a pleasant walk (or the Rainbow Bridge[1] for pet bereavement) and the imagination of the client will do the rest.

I developed this idea for a woman who had lost a child; in her case, when they met, I forward-paced the newborn and allowed the mother to see them as an older child to make conversation easier. You will, of course, have to tailor the meeting part of the script to suit your client's needs. It can be adapted for a child, adult, pet or anything else since, in this place, anyone lost is happy and fulfilled.

. . .

I would like you to imagine that you're on a walk to a place that you have never been to before. You walk along a path, and the uncertain haze of spring gently lifts to show, in the distance, lush green fields. Doves glide in the smooth sky, as their white feathers gently tickle the clouds and move them on their way, as if guided by a warm gentle breeze. The day is now cloudless, and the light blue sky pushes through, never to be hidden again. The light of the golden sun is pure and eternal; no cloud can hide its awesome warm rays as they gently warm your skin to a pleasant temperature. There is no pollen in the air, and you can take in the crisp, smooth air which fills your lungs and frees you from the rigmarole of the day-to-day.

You follow an orbital path that is around a still, cobalt-blue lake. Its reflections and lapping waves mirror the blue sky. The gentle movements catch your eye, and you relax with each wave as it is born, each grows and forms a smooth 'S' shape, then re-joins the perfectly formed basin as the waves gently lap against the shore.[2]

Your mind wanders, and your thoughts drift to your feet; the path gently supports your strides, and you feel the privilege of walking on untrodden terrain. The surface is spongy and light, and it makes walking a pleasure, and so easy. You travel at a good pace and notice a white Tholos[3] in the distance. It stands tall and proud, perfectly circular, as if it rests outside the tides of time.

You are drawn to this. As you move with ease it gets closer and closer and, before you realise it, you're halfway there. You notice the backdrop behind the Tholos has now become populated with moving colours that are lit with the sun's rays peeping over the trees. The sound of distant laughter can be heard, and this draws you closer still to the Tholos.

You approach the Tholos and see the tall, solid columns towering over you. The light peers through and illuminates a bench.

The bench, curved like a half moon, sits on the far side of the structure. It sits overlooking the fields and the dancing colours. You carefully enter, and as you do so, you feel the firmness of the marble floor. If it had not been for the colours in the background, you might never have noticed the Tholos and would have had no reason to venture towards it if you had passed by it. As you sit on the cushioned stone bench, overlooking the wavy colours, you are enveloped by a strong sense of freedom and happiness.

A figure in the distance breaks from the colours and moves towards you. The sounds of music reverberate off the columns of the building surrounding you in a pleasant choral harmony, and the sounds sweep through, charming your ear. As you listen to the music, that familiar presence comes your way. This is someone you know but who has fallen from sight. They are coming towards you slowly and calmly; you feel safe and secure as they move towards the seat and sit beside you. When you gaze at one another, you recognise that it is

[*insert the name of the individual who passed away.*]

Time is starting to slow. The sun gently saunters across the sky, and the wind softly drops from a waving of the grass to a gentle swaying of the pasture. There is plenty of time to enjoy the warm sunshine, as it encourages you to spend time with

[*insert the name of the individual who passed away.*]

This is a once-in-a-lifetime opportunity. We know that

[*insert the name of the individual who passed away*]

had gone before you had the chance to say everything to them. Now, here is your opportunity to say what you could not.

[*Add details here if you wish, by giving a description of the baby as a young child or adult or reminding them that the person is now whole and well.*]

See how they are as you remember them at their best; notice that, here, they are happy, free from pain and they accept what happened. They are ready to listen to your feelings, to help you through the healing process. Take your time, and convey everything you need to, as of this moment time is on your side. I am going to step away to keep this conversation private although I will be nearby if you need me. I have also seen someone here I would like to talk to, so please enjoy your conversation.

[*Saying you will give them privacy is designed to give the client reassurance that their conversation will not be overheard. Give as much time as they need, five minutes is often about right, but longer may be required, so be vigilant to the client's needs.]*

When you are ready to move on, and you have said everything that you need to, please signal by moving a finger or just saying you are ready.

Thank you. Now that you are ready to move on, you see

[insert the name of the individual who passed away]

move slowly and gently towards the colours. You see them happy, whole, and part of the fold. There is no pain, no suffering, only the ever-expanding light. You notice your feelings, and become aware that there has been a resolution, you feel calm and collected. Your vision returns to nature as you wish

[insert the name of the individual who passed away]

a fond farewell. Serenity, placidity, and tranquillity begin to spread through your body as your attention returns to nature. You notice as you return down the path, that time has caught up with itself, and you are now becoming aware of the warm sun rays of the afternoon, which are slowly declining into a summer's evening. The sky remains clear, to light the rest of the landscape, which is completely untouched, and completely filled with song. You hear birds in the background, and the subtle callings of a cuckoo can be heard in the distance. The lake meanders off into estuaries and you can follow them, parallel to the path, as you venture further outward.

You notice dry reeds, brittle spines, and the smells of the summer's evening, as the sun begins to tuck itself behind the horizon.

In a moment, soon, but not yet, we're going to revitalise, reawaken and re-engage with the conscious world. Take a moment to ready yourself and enjoy those pleasant happy feelings as well as the newfound calm and peace spread through you.

[Pause one minute before beginning your awakening process.]

The Author:

Brian Turner is a fully qualified and practising hypnotherapist and therapeutic supervisor. He is an accredited registrant of the National Hypnotherapy Society and also a member of the GHR. Before entering the world of hypnotherapy, Brian spent nine years in education in a variety of different roles, supporting and teaching individuals in a variety of settings.

Brian says, 'I have always been an active learner, and I've always sought to pass on my enthusiasm for learning in a variety of different subjects. I run my own, and jointly run, accredited CPD courses to actively pass on the learning bug and encourage others to seek new knowledge to better themselves in whatever profession may suit them; after all, I believe that education is something that someone is passionate about and leaving the world in a better place than they found it. As with any of my roles in providing therapeutic CPD education, I do not necessarily see myself as a provider but a facilitator to help individuals better themselves whilst maintaining the highest possible standards to give students the confidence to practice effectively in the therapeutic field.'

Brian is also the author of the book 'Lessons Learned in the Therapy Business', a reflection of the knowledge he has gathered over his years in practice.

OAK TREE

CAROL LIGHTOWLER

Personalisation:

A really nice metaphor which taps into a saying we all know – from little acorns great oaks grow. The acorn here is spoken of as 'she'. To help client identification it would be useful to change that to the pronoun the client applies to themselves.

It's ideal for clients who feel 'stuck' or feel afraid of new experiences and change.

Now, as you are relaxed and comfortable, your mind drifting or listening carefully to my words, I'm reminded of a story I used to know.

It was autumn, and a stout oak tree began to shed its cupped acorns onto the leaf-littered ground below. Squirrels scratched among the leaves, and scurried around, eating some of the acorns and storing others away in secret places at the foot of other trees.

But two acorns remained amongst the fallen leaves, which gradually lost their golden hue and became darker, turning into a rich, dark earthy-smelling substance, into which the acorns sank deeper.

The first acorn was fearful, worried about the changes which were happening. It dreamed of returning to the past, when it hung, safely swinging from a branch, high above the place where it now felt imprisoned. It held itself tight, hardening its shell for protection, holding itself secure, building a barrier against the changes that were happening. It told itself that, if only it could shut itself off from this strange new place, it would be fine.

The second acorn sank deeper and deeper among the leaves, which were becoming ever moister and a deeper, darker, brown. It was comfortable here, and though she didn't understand what was happening, she had a sense that everything would be fine. She settled down, snuggling into the dark softness, and dreamed of settling here, just knowing that this was where she needed to be for now. Things were changing, and she had faith.

Autumn turned to winter, and the ground became hard, both acorns remaining in the darkness below. The first acorn had shielded itself and felt secure, locked within its hard impenetrable shell. The second acorn felt herself unlocking in some way; something was changing, and she opened herself to the change. Winter turned into spring, and she opened up even further, sensing new energy inside. Feeling the need to ground herself, to hold herself steady in this ever-changing world, she sent down a white root which twisted and turned amongst the stones around her, finding a deep, rich place from which she could draw sustenance. At the same time, she felt herself bursting open, joyfully sending up a vibrant green shoot through the dark dampness into the clear bright daylight.

The first acorn held itself tightly closed, fearful of the world around.

Spring turned into summer, and the warmth of summer became the crispness of autumn. A young squirrel scratched deeply below the leaf litter and lifted up an old, dry acorn in its paws before sinking its teeth into the shrivelled shell whilst, nearby, an oak sapling looked on, its few leaves yellowing at the edges and falling to the ground. Feeling stable and securely rooted, the sapling knew that she could hold herself steady during the coming winter, and she dreamed of summer when she would unfold her bright serrated leaves and hold them proudly in the sunlight again, or securely through the raindrops, her trunk's girth expanding throughout her journey towards becoming the beautiful oak tree that she was always meant to be.

The Author:

Carol Lightowler initially trained as an integrative counsellor, drawing from several therapeutic traditions to develop individual therapeutic models for each client. She graduated with distinction in 2007 and has since worked as a counsellor in a variety of settings. She views her work as primarily rooted in intersubjectivity but, increasingly, it has been necessary to integrate therapeutic techniques into this relationally based work to work in a more solution-focused way.

She began to integrate creative visualisation into her practice during initial training, and later discovered Jon Kabat Zinn's work on the use of mindfulness and started to explore how mindfulness might be used to benefit both herself and her clients.

She was wary of the possibility of the re-traumatisation of certain clients and began to research new tools to integrate within her practice. Whilst CBT approaches offered something useful, she found that many clients were unable to reflect upon, or re-frame their experience whilst experiencing high levels of emotional arousal. After undertaking a 'Rewind' course, a client mentioned that hypnotherapy had been very helpful in releasing negative images, and Carol also decided to learn more about that.

Whilst Carol still regards herself as an integrative psychotherapeutic counsellor, after successfully completing a course in clinical hypnotherapy with Debbie Waller she is now able to integrate hypnotherapy within her psychotherapeutic work.

Carol draws from various traditions to offer clients what is most useful to them and feels hypnotherapy offers an additional tool in supporting clients.

Carol's website is www.clcounselling.co.uk

THE PRINCESS AND THE ROPE

AUTHOR: LYN PALMER

Personalisation:

A traditional fairy story approach here, about a princess and the trouble she got into with a magical rope. It was originally developed for a client whose motivation to complete a task was inhibited by insecurity and negative internal dialogue. It's also great for 'imposter syndrome' and any client who lacks confidence or motivation because they don't believe in themselves.

The princess in the story often thinks of herself as 'silly', which is not necessarily a word you want to use about your client! Listen to their descriptions and metaphors. The words they use about themselves for not getting things done might be lazy, daft, fearful, or any one of many other negative labels. Make sure you substitute this for 'silly' in the story and adapt the words around your chosen descriptor to make it fit.

And I'd make it a prince rather than a princess, if your client identifies as male.

Your situation reminds me of the story I once heard about a princess. She was out playing by herself one day, and she came across a box labelled 'wizardry rope'.

She looked inside and saw a thick piece of rope, but she couldn't work out what was 'wizardry' about it. She played with it for a while, but still could not work out what was different about this particular piece of rope. She tied it around her hands but, once she had done this, she realised that she couldn't untie it. The princess thought that she might get in trouble for playing with the magical rope so, when she went back to the castle, she hid her hands and went straight to bed.

The next morning, she thought that when the maid came to get her up, she would see the rope and untie it. However, the maid didn't say anything about the rope, and the princess didn't want to mention it first, because she thought that everyone would say that she had been silly to tie it around her hands.

When she went to breakfast, the King and Queen didn't mention the rope, and the same thing happened when she went to school; none of the teachers or the other children mentioned the rope. She soon came to realise that what was magical about the rope was that it was only visible to her, to everyone else it was invisible. She thought to herself, 'As no one can see the rope except me, if I don't tell anyone about it, then no one will think I'm silly, only I will know.'

As she grew up, the princess got used to finding ways to do things with an invisible rope around her hands. In fact, she did things so well that no one ever guessed that she was constrained by an invisible rope. The King often went off visiting foreign lands, and one day he returned with great news for the princess; he had found a prince in the next kingdom that he thought would be a perfect match for her. The prince wanted to know more about all the local princesses before he chose his bride and, to have the opportunity for an audience with him, all she had to do was write him a letter in her own fair hand, telling him all about herself.

The King was very excited about this and encouraged the princess to start writing a letter straight away: audiences with the prince were going to be happening soon. But the princess became very anxious. She really wanted to write the letter, because the prince sounded like a perfect match for her, but every time she thought about it or tried to start, she worried that she would never be good enough because of the constraints of the invisible rope.

The princess kept making excuses as to why she couldn't write the letter, until one day the King came to see her to explain that there were only two weeks left now to get it done. The princess was still feeling very anxious but decided that enough was enough, she would finally have to tell the King about the invisible rope. She was fed up with it holding her back.

She summoned all her courage and told the King about the rope that had constrained her since she was a child. As soon as she did this, something amazing happened! The rope suddenly became visible to the King.

As soon as the King saw the rope he said kindly, 'Why on earth have you been wearing this all these years?' The princess told him how she thought that she had been silly to wind the rope around her hands in the first place and she didn't want everyone else to think the same thing about her.

The King was sad that the princess had been constrained like this and told her that she certainly was not silly. He commanded that the rope should be removed immediately.

When it was, the princess took hold of the rope and flung it into the fire. She felt such a wonderful feeling of freedom as the smoke from the burning rope rose higher and higher away from her, reducing the rope to nothing but ashes.

The princess no longer felt silly and realised that in fact she never had been. She had just been afraid of what other people might think, so she hid her real feelings, and her limitations, and tried to manage around them instead of asking for help.

Now she felt carefree, confident, happy and self-assured. She started to write her letter to the prince straight away, telling him all about herself, her experiences of being a princess in her kingdom and how she would like to come and meet with him in his kingdom.

Once she had posted her letter, in good time to meet the

deadline, the princess reflected on what had happened. She thought to herself, 'Although I would like to meet the prince, that's not the most important thing. I've sent my letter and now it's up to him to decide if he would like to meet me or not. Even if we do meet, there's no guarantee that we will be the perfect match for each other, but what is important is that I have finally rid myself of the rope, and I am free to do whatever I want.'

The princess felt proud of what she had achieved and had a new sense of assured confidence that showed in everything she did. She knew that, without the rope, she could be herself, she had nothing to hide, and she had enough confidence in herself to make her own choices in life, whether she married the prince, or did something else completely different.

The Author:

Lyn Palmer says, 'I have always been interested in people; what makes us do the things we do; react in the way we react, and how we connect with others. I love people-watching, not in a judgemental way, but in observation of what makes us who we are. We are such individuals, each with our own point of view, and I think it's fascinating to gain an understanding of others' perspectives.

Having worked for corporate businesses all my working life, in 2014 I moved into a coaching role, which cemented my belief that I enjoy helping people on their journey of growth and progress.

I had previously undertaken some hypnotherapy for myself and eventually decided to take the leap to become a hypnotherapist. I qualified in 2019 and subsequently set up my own private practice.

I work with clients experientially on a person-centred basis, utilising various methods of hypnotherapy that combine to work for the client. My work incorporates working with parts, carrying out regressions, both this life and past life, gestalt therapy, and forward pacing. I find that in any of these areas, weaving in a metaphor can have a strong impact because the subconscious mind will relate it to the client's own perspective and, therefore, they gain insight and change which is very individual to them.

I love being able to help people to help themselves to become stronger people, leading happier lives.'

Lyn's website is www.withyouinmind.info

THE TAILOR AND THE GLOVEMAKER

AUTHOR: RACHEL GOTH

Personalisation:

This one reminds me very strongly of Hans Christian Andersen's stories because it's about craftsmen (although the obligatory fairy-tale princess acts as a catalyst for their story). It has a lot to say about perfectionism, control, and over-planning. There is, of course, nothing wrong with wanting to do your best, but aiming for excellence is better than obsessing over small details and needing perfection every time!

I would adjust the genders of the friends in the tale to match the one the client identifies with, to help them get into the story and, if they have a creative hobby or job, you could even rewrite parts to give the tailor a different job which matches the client's interests.

There were once two friends, who had recently graduated from their apprenticeships in tailoring and fashion. Both dreamed of having amazing careers and making their fortune.

One day, they each received a telegram from the palace, inviting them to create something for the princess's birthday. Along with the other craftspeople of the city, they would be invited to an exclusive gathering where they could give her their gifts in person.

Both the friends were beside themselves with excitement, this could mean a lot for their careers. Neither of them, however, had the means to spend a lot of money on materials. So, what fine gifts could they make?

One of the friends decided to make the princess a pair of gloves. The other friend scoffed at the idea of making something so small and decided to design a coat, the most exquisite garment the land had ever seen.

The glovemaker questioned the tailor about how he could afford such an extravagant gift, but the tailor simply chastised her for her lack of ambition and would hear no more about it.

Each of them was allowed one fitting with the princess, which they made the most of, scribbling notes and double-checking their measurements. They now had three weeks to make their creations and present them to the princess at her birthday party.

The glovemaker set to work immediately, creating a pattern, buying the best quality material she could afford and beginning work. Meanwhile, the tailor took their time scouring the kingdom for the finest materials that he could not afford so he had to borrow from here, there and everywhere. But the tailor wasn't worried at all. He was convinced that the kudos alone from his fabulous creation would repay the debt tenfold.

Finally, the tailor had gathered all the luxurious fabrics and adornments he wished to use. That night he lay in bed imagining the wonderful coat he would create. How fine it would feel to touch, how beautiful it would be to behold. But a seed of doubt began to grow. What if the measurements were not precise enough? What if they were a millimetre too small, too wide, or too tall?

The glovemaker awoke very early to the tailor hammering at her door to share his worries. The glovemaker did her best to soothe her friend and told him not to worry, but the tailor could not shake the thought of embarrassing himself in front of the finest craftspeople in the kingdom.

So, the very next morning, following a sleepless night, the tailor arrived at the palace to see the princess. He insisted an extra fitting was crucial as this was going to be the greatest coat in the world, but the guards only laughed, and the tailor was turned away.

However, an aide to the princess who was passing by overheard the tailor and relayed the incident to her. Intrigued by what she heard the princess sent for the tailor.

Over the moon, the tailor came straight away. He described the coat to the princess as the most beautiful creation of purest wool, lined with the most stunning silk. Decorated with rare, hand-carved buttons made by the reclusive monks of a far-off isle. Smooth as butter, bejewelled, and sparkling with fine threads. Even the coat's aroma would be rich and warming, a treat for the senses. It would fit like a glove, hugging her every curve and she would be the envy of every other royal. Impressed, the princess agreed to a new fitting.

The tailor carefully took the princess's measurements again, double and triple-checking before hurrying home to work well into the night.

Word soon got around about the legendary coat the tailor was making and people clamoured at the tailor's door with orders. But the tailor was busy. He had no time for them and told them impatiently that they'd have to wait. Meanwhile, the glovemaker had made good progress on her gloves and decided to make some other accessories to sell at the local market.

The princess's birthday arrived, and the city's craftspeople lined up to give her their presents. The princess received many fine gifts, including from the glovemaker. The tailor sneered at the lack of detail and the inferiority of the material, but the glovemaker was happy that she'd done her best with the resources and time she had. The princess herself was delighted with the gloves, exclaiming they were just what she needed for the coming winter.

When it came to the tailor's turn, he begged the princess for a little more time, and promised that the coat would be all the more opulent for it. The disappointed princess reluctantly agreed.

The following day, the tailor arrived again at the palace to ask for another fitting, just to be quite sure the coat would be perfect.

But, of course, after all the festivities the princess was a little bloated. So, when the tailor checked the princess's measurements, they had changed ever so slightly. The tailor took the new measurements and set about adapting the pattern.

Of course, as is liable to happen, a couple of weeks later, when the tailor called yet again for a final check, the princess's measurements had gone back to normal. The tailor insisted the coat would now be too big even though it was just a few millimetres. The princess tried to reassure the tailor it would be fine, but the tailor insisted on making more adjustments.

As autumn turned to winter, the princess was often seen wearing her new gloves. The glovemaker began to receive commissions from across the land and was building a good reputation.

But as different festivities came and went, the princess's measurements fluctuated ever so slightly, invisible to the naked eye, yet each time the tailor measured again, insisting on making further adjustments.

By the time the glovemaker had made enough money to buy her own workshop and was building quite a reputation, the tailor's waiting list of clients slowly had but surely ebbed away. The glovemaker offered to give the tailor some work but he was too busy. Besides, he scoffed at what he saw as the glovemaker's inferior products. They would pale in comparison when the princess donned her magnificent coat.

Winter turned to spring and the princess didn't have the heart to turn away the tailor, so she continued to allow the fittings, even though she'd long since given up hope of ever receiving the legendary coat. As the tailor tucked and pinned, the princess's mind drifted away to foreign climes. In particular, to the desert island of the reclusive monks who the tailor told her carved the rare and beautiful buttons which would adorn the coat.

Then, one day, the excited tailor demanded the glovemaker accompany him to the palace for an audience with the princess, declaring that the coat was ready at last.

For the glovemaker, their gift for the princess was now a footnote in their career, they'd moved on to many other and more lucrative commissions. But this was make or break for the tailor, he'd sunk every penny he had and more besides into this coat. It was the only piece he'd worked on since graduating from his apprenticeship, and his whole reputation and future career depended on it. The tailor still believed that pouring everything into the coat had been the right decision and he wanted his friend the glovemaker to be there to see his triumph.

And it was indeed the finest coat in the kingdom, the princess exclaimed. Soft to the touch, the smoothest silk lining, and detail the likes of which she had never seen. It fitted her like a second skin, the lines followed her body perfectly, giving a sense of grace to her every movement, leaving not a millimetre where a cold breeze might dare to creep. The tailor was elated.

But a sadness crept across the princess, as she slowly unbuttoned the coat. She told the tailor she was travelling to a far-off land. Inspired by her daydreams during their many fittings, she was going on a pilgrimage to seek out the reclusive monks who had carved the exquisite buttons on her coat. The desert isles of their home would be far too hot for such warm clothing. The tailor's heart sank.

But then, the princess brightened as she called to her aide. She bade the woman try on the garment. The tailor looked on aghast as the young woman put on the exquisite creation. She was of a similar age to the princess, a little shorter and slightly narrower. All that time wasted, perfecting every inch, for it now to be transformed into an ill-fitting covering for a maid! The tailor saw his reputation in tatters before him. How could he ever hold his head up high again? The tailor turned away in shame.

The glovemaker, who had been silently watching, patted the tailor on the back and said, 'It still does the job, my friend'. And before the tailor could reply the princess clasped her hands together in glee.

The tailor followed the princess's gaze to her maid twirling around in her new coat, a broad smile spread across her face. She had never owned anything so magnificent. 'Well, I suppose it will keep her warm' the tailor thought. Which, of course, is the purpose of a coat.

The princess was delighted to see her aide so happy and asked the tailor if he could make coats for the rest of the staff in time for winter. The tailor worried that the fine adornments alone would take weeks, but the maid assured him that, lovely as those decorations were, they would only get dirty during her duties. And the tailor conceded, if only to himself, that, for practical purposes, those details were, indeed, unnecessary.

Then the tailor argued that there was no more fine silk to make the linings. But the glovemaker offered the tailor some of their cotton. And the tailor had to agree that cotton would be a more practical material for a work garment. 'Think of it now,' the glovemaker said. 'Instead of tailoring for one princess, you'll be tailor to the entire royal staff'. And the tailor couldn't help but smile to himself.

And so, the tailor began to work on a plan to design a practical coat for the working members of the court. Something he could make quickly and that would do the job. And whenever the tailor was tempted to get carried away, obsessing over fine details, the glovemaker would give him a look, and the tailor would laugh and refocus on the important parts of the job until it was all done, and everyone at the palace was smart and warm for the winter.

The Author:

Rachel Goth is a trained master coach and hypnotherapist, who specialises in helping coaches, therapists and teachers learn to love their voice, so they can share their message without having to change the way they speak.

She knows first-hand what it's like learning to use your voice for your business, show up as yourself on social media and create recordings for your clients. She now helps her clients to do the same by helping them move from disliking their voices to becoming confident in the way they sound.

Through a combination of 1:1 coaching, and practical exercises, Rachel helps her clients establish a new positive belief in their voice, so they feel confident being themselves and sharing their message. Within a couple of weeks, her clients are confidently recording their own meditations, creating courses, and ad-libbing their social media videos with ease.

Find out more at rachelgoth.com

YOU ARE A GENIE

AUTHOR: DAVID SEAR

Personalisation:

This unusual journey through the land of Oz to Aladdin's lamp is a magical take on the idea of the inner advisor. It is designed to help *your client make decisions with confidence. The story should give them a clearer understanding of their decision-making process, and the positive, natural way in which this happens should also create a sense of calmness and self-control.*

It's a good idea, before starting, to have talked about at least one specific decision the client is facing, and the options they are trying to choose between. This makes it much easier to personalise the part of the session where they ask their genie for help.

Read this slowly, especially when you get to the part where you are suggesting questions. Give them time for the answers to pop into their minds.

How many times each day do you need to make a decision? Some are small, almost insignificant choices to make, for example, the choice about what you are going to eat, your outfit for the day or what to watch on television. As we know, we can choose our own path and some of your decisions can feel much more difficult to make. Some life choices are so important, that you cannot just dive in. Test your imagination now and let it run free as I guide you through this decision-making process.

Picture a scene in your head, as we go deep into your imagination and begin to get really creative. Just like in the Wizard of Oz, the first image I want you to see is a beautiful, twisting, yellow brick road. As you look ahead, the road winds into the distance and you cannot see its conclusion. Think about how wide the road is. The sky is blue, and the sun is shining, but I want you to complete this view and add the surroundings on both sides of the road. You may decide on a grassed verge, or maybe bigger still, an enchanted forest. There could be farmer's fields containing livestock, or maybe you can see crops growing in the sunlight. Whatever you decide, you feel calm, happy, and a tinge of excitement as you follow the yellow brick road! This is a long journey, so take your time. The road winds left and right and, at the same time, climbs quite steeply before dropping back down again. All the time, take notice of the ever-changing scenery around you on the left and on the right.

And you can continue to make this imagining strong and powerful, in whatever way is exciting and positive for you.

Eventually, as you continue to stay focused on this wonderful journey, the yellow bricks come to an end, and you find yourself in a clearing. This circular area is dusty on the ground and the entire space is grey in colour. The sun is disappearing, and the light is fading. Just ahead of you is a golden-coloured oil lamp. You think to yourself, 'How weird it is to see this object just sat there by itself'.

It looks ancient, it has a few dents here and there, but it's intact and has an elegant appearance with some pretty finishing flourishes, like ornate engravings on the lid and spout. See yourself now walking towards the lamp, bending down, and picking the item up. It is much bigger than you imagined.

Holding it up, at head height, in front of you, the delicate and intricate patterns can be examined. It is obvious that this is a special lamp. Memories of fairy tales, childhood fables and fantasy stories fill your brain, but we now concentrate on the seriousness and clear and concise messages that this lamp can portray. The lamp may give you indications of positivity. You feel privileged to hold it in the palms of your hands. It feels so old, as you inspect it further.

Just like in the story, give the lamp a little rub on the side. With a puff of smoke, a purple haze shoots out of the spout of the lamp. The foggy area clears, and you see something remarkable standing in front of you – a genie!

Think to yourself exactly what your genie looks like. How tall are they? What are they wearing? Maybe they are sporting ancient silks or draped in gold jewellery and gemstones? Have they got pointed shoes? Their clothing is probably colourful and glamorous. Concentrate on the full view of your genie from head to toe, take in their presence and authority, and be in awe of this sight. Hold this vision in your mind.

Focus now on the face of the figure that stands before you. This face looks a lot like you. Almost like a clone of your being, or a face-shaped mirror ahead of you. Is this just a version of yourself? Your creative side? The part of you that makes those decisions we talked about, figuring out the results of certain scenarios? Is this the part of your mind that helps you come to conclusions or guides you down the correct road, whether yellow or any other colour?

Look into the eyes on this face. A face you can trust. Look at the genie's mouth and you know that, deep in your mind, you trust the words that come from it. See the honesty from those eyes. Absorb and study the sight of this face.

This genie is not like the one in the children's story. There are no three wishes. They do not exist here. This is your own personal genie, whom you can visit anytime you please. Your genie will always give you honesty and loyalty. So, how can your genie help you?

You can ask your genie anything you wish. Whether it is something small, or a situation that could possibly be life-changing, utilise your genie. Remember, you will always get an honest answer. When you ask your genie a question in your mind, stay focused on him or her. When you get a response, it may well be in the form of an indication. For example, you may well receive a nod or a shake of the head. You may get a reply by way of a hand gesture and, yes, sometimes this gesture may be rude! You may get a smile or a frown when you ask your query. On the other hand, you may get involved in a full-blown conversation with your genie.

It is important that you take in all the information from your visit. Trust in the detail. Believe in your genie.

[*The following two paragraphs can be altered to reflect the client's own decisions and the choices they are facing, which you will know about through your intake conversation.*]

When we talk about life-changing questions, what exactly do we mean? You may have come to a crossroads in your career and you're seeking advice regarding an employment offer. There might be a decision to make that involves your family, delicate options which affect them as much as you. Moving home is something that affects most of us in our lifetime. This can be stressful, but are you doing the right thing? Do you want another child? Are you ready to retire? Can you afford that dream holiday? Choices that we must make all the time as we go about our daily business.

Ask your genie fun questions too. What to wear at a party, what colour to dye your hair, Christmas gift ideas and many others where you have multiple options. You could say that this is almost like talking to yourself by looking in the mirror, but creating this genie gives more clarity and thought to the decisions that you make.

Take in and absorb all the information relayed to you from your genie. Take your time and thank him or her at the end of your visit. Remember, your visits are unlimited. Always bid a fond farewell before making that journey back on the long and winding yellow brick road. As you make this journey home, give yourself time to ponder the results of your visit.

Remember that you can visit your genie at any time, just by

finding somewhere safe and comfortable to relax, where you won't be interrupted for a while, and imagining yourself back on that yellow brick road, finding the lamp.

It's important to be aware of the results of your visits. Give yourself time after each visit to think about the results, as sometimes you have more than one choice to make. Trust in yourself and that gut feeling. Trust your genie.

[*Follow this with some future pacing, imagining the future with the decision confidently made, the client and others happy with the outcome etc before reorienting the client.*]

The Author:

David Sear says of himself: 'I have always been a people person. Providing great service and helping people has always been important to me, whatever my job role was. Over the past ten years, I have been interested in alternative therapies and treatments, and I found myself specifically attracted to hypnotherapy. From there, I studied a wide range of hypnosis treatments, and I became a fully qualified and accredited hypnotherapist. I now have a practice in York.'

Copyright note: 'You are the genie' was first published in 'Open Your Mind: Visualisations – Create A Better Life' by David Sear, ISBN 1838197303, which is available on Amazon. It is included here with the kind permission of the author. It was presented originally for self-help and the wording has been adjusted to allow you to use it with clients.

CHAPTER SIX

HOBBIES, JOBS, AND INTERESTS

An extremely effective way to make a metaphor meaningful is to use one based on ideas and themes that are already familiar to your client and, in this chapter, we have stories that specifically talk about hobbies, interests and even jobs that clients might have.

A few of the metaphors in other chapters might be relevant to clients' interests too, for example:

- Any of those set in the countryside or on a beach for those who like walking or holidays.
- Boris and the Wheel (in Mini Metaphors) for those who like animals.
- Aromas and Rhythms (in Kaleidoscope) for those who like flowers, aromatherapy or music.
- Weeds (in clearing metaphors) for those who like their gardens

THE CAR

AUTHOR: BARBARA GRAVIL

Personalisation:

D*efinitely one for car enthusiasts, since it mentions liking the smell of oil and petrol!*

This metaphor is very much about seeing hidden qualities, healing from neglect or abuse and gaining the confidence to enjoy life again. It's great for those who feel bombarded by life, with everything being thrown at them from all directions, and who feel that they lack the ability to be there for family members (like children) who rely on them.

You can adapt this by ensuring that the model and make of the car are the client's dream car, if you know it, or at least their favourite colour. Or, if you prefer to make the client an observer, you could change it to a third-person point of view and have them watch their favourite TV car show presenter discover and work on the car.

Imagine that you are standing in a street. It might be a familiar street, or one that you don't know, created by your wonderful imagination. Take a look around, and notice what's there.

In the distance, you notice a garage, with its door slightly ajar.

Walking towards it, you step inside, breathing in the smell of oil and petrol that you so love.

[The next sentence assumes the client has experience working on old cars; if not, you can replace it with something more relevant, like 'You are immediately reminded of your dream and ambition to work on old cars.']

You are immediately transported back to those happy days, when you would don your overalls and spend many hours working on your car.

Closing your eyes, you breathe in that smell of happiness, of that happy place and that feeling of security and contentment.

Opening your eyes, you notice the most beautiful car. It would have been majestic in its former glory, but now, it's faded grandeur, apologetic. Neglected and alone. You walk around it, noting its paintwork, shabby and dull. The bodywork is covered in dust.

Tentatively stroking its panel, you open the driver's door. It creaks slowly open; it seems careful not to cause offence. Knowing it has been abused and neglected. Regretful to find itself here in this sorry state. But *you* can see it. You can see its beauty and splendour. You know it's all still there. Lurking. Waiting. Hoping.

Daring to seat yourself in the driver's seat, you feel the old leather of the steering wheel in your palms and notice the gentle cracking of the seats. Closing your eyes, you breathe in that mixture of old leather, oil, and petrol, breathing out concern and insecurity. Just enveloping yourself in happiness and hope, with a deep knowing that all will be well. You can feel the seats cocooning you, safely protecting you, as you will protect it.

Just like a child about to blossom, reaching out for a hand to guide and steady them along the way. You are there, but you have to let them fall. They fall and they pick themselves up. Moving forward, not glancing back. Standing tall, facing the world. Just as you are facing the world. Proud, straight and tall. Proud of yourself and proud of them. Knowing that some things cannot be changed, but they *can* be dealt with.

This lovely car never lost its worth. It just got hidden away for a while. Waiting until the time was right. Well, now you're here. You see what others cannot. Your empathy is commendable. If others knew what you knew, they would applaud you.

But less – less of this! You have a job to do, and this amazing car is relying on you. Looking to you. Waiting for you. It appears broken, but you know that it can be mended. Mended with tweaks that will enhance its performance. Growling it back into life. Purring along its journey.

Picking up passengers along the way. Giving them, too, direction. They have a lot to learn before they reach their destination. They will thank you for your help. They will fondly remember it as they journey themselves. You may carpool, travel with a friend by your side, enjoy the conversation and share the views. Enjoying the familiar companionship. There are many paths leading to your destination. Enjoy your journey. Notice and appreciate the beauty you see along the way.

You know what you have to do. You pity the neglecters, and you journey on. You accept the neglect, with a deep knowing that such things can be mended and will be even better than before. Shinier, brighter, greater than before. Yet still remaining reliable and in control, with the deepest, deepest, feeling of contentment and security.

Now.

The oil has been changed.

The timing belt has been adjusted.

The leather is waxed and well cared for.

The paintwork is primped and polished.

The tyres are pumped-up.

The carpets are cleaned and freshly hoovered.

The car is re-fuelled, and its service was long overdue. But it is now complete.

And now, the time is right. The day is here. The car is restored and enhanced, leading others with her bright, shiny lights.

Who knows what is in the distance? Who can tell?

But you are excited – looking forward to the journey.

Rallying the bumps and strains along the way. Changing gear to gain control. Remember that you do not need to journey alone.

Yes. You're ready. The time is right.

The Author:

Barbara Gravil qualified through the Royal Academy as a piano teacher over thirty-five years ago and it was this that led her to seek the assistance of hypnotherapy for performance nerves. She was amazed at how much it helped. Shortly after this, her mum became ill and needed strong pain relief. Barbara had a hypnotherapy recording made for her and was shocked (and relieved) at the effectiveness of hypnotherapy once again. This sparked a lifelong interest.

Over time, Barbara noticed that some of her most talented students became highly self-critical and increasingly wary of recitals and milestone practical examinations. Some would be about to audition for highly acclaimed educational establishments, when they would be overcome with anxiety. Within a short space of time, a few of her pupils tried hypnotherapy and their composure was restored. That was it – she needed to know more!

Fast forward to a taster day with YHT and she was well and truly hooked. Barbara now informs her students of her training, and her ability to offer help with anxiety alongside musical tuition. Her particular interest in the alleviation of performance nerves has led her to work with all forms of anxiety. After helping friends and family cope with various health issues, she also found herself led towards helping cancer patients along their often-difficult journey.

As a sidenote, Barbara is pleased with the side-effect hypnotherapy has had on her dog, Frank. He has never been calmer and has decided to leave the cat-chasing behind him!

www.barbaragravil.com

DETECTIVE WORK

AUTHOR: CATHERINE DAYCOCK

Personalisation:

I doubt many of your clients will be real-life detectives, but they have more than likely seen crime shows on television, or perhaps they enjoy reading murder mysteries. This taps into the Sherlockian instinct in us all to hunt for clues and discover solutions to help resolve the client's presenting issue.

There are plenty of questions and alternatives in the opening paragraphs, all of which help the client to imagine the scene in their own way. Read these slowly, leaving pauses between each one so they have time to answer in their heads.

If your client really is a crime fiction buff, find out what kind they prefer (cosy stuff like Murder She Wrote, hard-boiled like Raymond Chandler, or police procedurals from James Patterson) and adapt the setting accordingly. Or ask who their favourite fictional detective is and introduce that person working alongside them on the crime board, helping with the case.

I'd like you to imagine that you find yourself in front of a door. You know instinctively that, when you open the door, you will find yourself in the office of a detective. Look at the door: is it an old, heavy wooden door? A new modern one? Perhaps it's a thin door from an office block in the '70s. Or maybe something completely different.

When you are ready, you open the door. Possibly, it opens easily, or it might be locked and require a key from a large keychain. Do you have to swipe to enter, or tap a code into a keypad beside the door? Now do whatever you have to and open the door.

It is now open, and you step inside and look around. Is the office big or small? Does it have any windows? Is it cluttered and piled high with files and paperwork?

Maybe it is neat and well organised, with everything neatly filed away in filing cabinets. Or perhaps it is sleekly designed with minimal furniture with everything you need stored on the computer on the desk.

However it looks, go and find yourself a seat at the desk. As you get comfortable in the chair, you take a look at what is on the desk.

To your surprise and delight, you see your name on the name plaque on the desk, 'Detective

[*insert the client's full name*]',

and you realise that this is your office, that you are the detective who works here! So, you have another look around the room. You are eager to see more, to find out what kind of detective you are, and what your assignment might be.

Glancing around the room, you pick up on the clues. Is it a detective agency and you are a private investor like Sam Spade? Or is the room full of beautiful ornate furniture and books, the office of an intelligent and calculating detective like Sherlock Holmes or Jessica Fletcher? Perhaps it is the office of a dogged detective like Columbo or Vera Stanhope, or maybe one of the meticulous modern investigators from CSI, who use DNA and forensics to solve the crime.

Whichever it is, you know that you are ready to take on the next assignment and solve the mystery. And, instinctively, you know that something special is going to occur – something that will answer an important question in your life or show you the direction you need to take next. At this stage, you are not sure what it will be, but you trust your instincts, and you know it's time to put your detective cap on, figuratively (or maybe even literally!) speaking.

Looking around the room, you now notice (if you didn't before) that there is a large empty board on one side of the room – your 'crime board'. So, you get up from where you were sitting behind the desk and make your way over to the board.

What does your investigation board look like? Is it a cork board with a box of drawing pins, or a white board with magnets and marker pens? Perhaps the board is more modern and is clear glass or Perspex? Whatever your board looks like, step back from it and take a good look. There is a title attached to the top, signifying the question or problem to be solved.

Can you already see what it says? If it's not clear, turn away from the board for a moment and take a deep breath, let yourself relax down even further, then turn back to the board and read what is there. What does it say? You may need to go deeper into your mind and ask yourself, 'What am I seeking? What am I looking for? What is the question that I want to answer today?' And when you do this, find that the question just pops into your mind. Once you have the question, nod to let me know.

[*Wait for a nod from the client.*]

Now, it's time to get all the important and relevant characters out on the board. Without trying too hard to remember everyone you think should be on there, just trust yourself and find a folder or a large manila envelope on the desk beside you. Open it up, pull out the photos and place them any way you see fit onto your board. Don't forget to include a picture of yourself if that is relevant. You might wish to place them all in a line, so everyone has equal status, or maybe you prefer to place them from top to bottom, to create a hierarchy showing who takes priority in the situation you're thinking about.

When you are happy with the order and arrangement of the main characters, you can open the other file or envelope that is on the desk. This time, you find an array of photos, pictures, maps, newspaper clippings – anything that represents elements of the question you want to answer. You can place these in whichever order you like, you can move them about, rearrange the board, make some larger if they hold more importance, or smaller if you find that if, on reflection, they are of less importance.

Take a few moments to find all the relevant pieces and find the right arrangement to help lay out the problem in visual form in front of you. Visualising everything in this way can help you see issues more clearly – it can help you identify the important and the less important aspects. As you sort through, you may decide to throw some of the images away if you realise that they hold very little significance or are, in fact, just a distraction from getting to the true solution.

You may find that other things come to mind that you haven't originally put on the board. That's fine, just find an object or image to represent those things and add them to your board, putting them in the appropriate place to start to make sense of their significance and meaning. I will be quiet for a few moments to allow you to do what you need to do, so please give me a nod when you've finished.

[*Wait for a nod from the client.*]

Now, you can take your whiteboard marker, or some pins and red string – whatever you have that suits your choice of investigation board – and start to link the various items on your board to each other, or highlight some areas over others, anything you need to do to help you solve the mystery.

Are the solutions starting to fall into place? Or is something blocking you? If so, what do you need to do to help the solution become clear?

Do you need to go to the crime scene? Watch the CCTV? See it from different angles?

You can do anything to help you to get to grips with the issue.

Maybe you need to interview the witnesses to see what others think and feel about your possible solutions, especially if they are going to be affected. Or, maybe, you just need to stand back from your investigation board and view it from another perspective.

As you do this, perhaps you realise that some things need to be altered. Maybe things need to be added or removed. Or just moved around to a different position, to allow you to gain a different viewpoint to assess and reassess all the different elements. I will be quiet for a few moments to allow you to do what needs to be done and to reflect on what the evidence is telling you. The solution should begin to float up to you from the board, or maybe it will suddenly pop into your mind, as if it came out of nowhere. Whatever way it happens, just nod to let me know you have found the solution.

[*Wait for a nod from the client.*]

Thank you – well done.

The final step is to check that the solution you have found is the correct one. If you're a private detective, you are your own client today, so check with all the other parts of you that will be affected. Or, if you have one, you can take your solution to the Chief, the Commanding Officer, or the Senior Investigating Officer, and see if they are happy with it.

[*Wait for a nod from the client and go to *. If you don't get a nod after a reasonable time, add the following suggestion.*]

If they are happy, you are ready and you should give me a nod. But, if not, you may need to go back and check the investigation board for something you have missed, or look at the problem again from a different perspective and allow a different solution to emerge.

[*Guide your client through the steps again if needed, until you get a positive affirmation that they have found the best solution.*]

*That's great. You have done brilliantly. Once you have found the best solution, the answer to your question will suddenly become clear. It may even seem so obvious that you're surprised you didn't see it before!

Take a moment to congratulate yourself on finding this solution, and then take the first, positive step towards achieving the solution. Just one small step, whatever that might be. Maybe resolving to speak to a specific person, or to take a particular action. Whatever it is, make a promise to yourself now that you will do it as soon as possible. And when you have decided on your first action, and made yourself that promise, give me a nod.

[*Wait for a nod from the client.*]

That's brilliant. You have done an excellent job. In a moment I will ask you to return to full awareness, and you will bring back with you all your newfound wisdom and solutions, ready to apply them to your life.

The Author:

Catherine Daycock says: 'I originally gained a degree in Criminology and Sociology and a Masters in Cultural Policy and Management, then went to work in the Financial Industry. So, it was a real departure to leave all that and retrain in hypnotherapy and NLP. I am so glad that I took that plunge, as it is a really rewarding and interesting career! I have my Diploma in Hypnotherapy, one in NLP, specialist diplomas in Gastric Band Hypnosis and Smoking Cessation, and am currently working towards my Diploma in Advanced Hypnotherapy.

I'm a single mum with two boys. Other than hypnotherapy, I am obsessed with True Crime – documentaries, books, and podcasts! I also enjoy crafts (when I get the chance) and have started gardening in the last couple of years so, in the summer, I try to get the entire front of my house covered in flowers!

For many years I have really struggled with anxiety and panic attacks. It got so bad in 2012 that I was unable to work, go anywhere or do anything. It was a struggle to even go to the local shop. Whilst

I didn't go to a hypnotherapist to help with this (oh, I wish I had known then what I know now!) it has given me a very real understanding of how debilitating such an issue can be, but also the knowledge that I can help my clients and there is light at the end of the tunnel.'

PERFECT FIT

AUTHOR: JOANNE AINLEY

Personalisation:

T his metaphor is about working with uncertainty, and it is
especially suitable if that comes from past negative influences and
labels.

Before using it, you'll need to identify three things: some family
members or friends from the client's support network; a place or situation
where the client wants to change their current feelings or behaviour; and
one or more negative experiences from the past whose influence they wish
to reduce.

The metaphor refers to sitting at 'your desk at work', but this could
easily be changed to match the client's specific working environment, for
example if they work outside or don't use a desk. The author has used
jigsaws here, but the basic framework will also adapt for use with other
creative hobbies such as mosaics or decoupage etc.

Imagine sitting down at your desk at work. It looks completely
familiar, with all your personal things in their usual places and
close at hand where you'd expect to see them.

Now, imagine noticing something new on your desk: a flat,

rectangular box that isn't usually there. It's the sort of box that could have a board game in it, and you might expect to see a cheerful picture on the front, perhaps showing people playing the game and enjoying it. But your box doesn't have a picture on the front, so you gently pick it up and shake it. It's not heavy but you can hear the contents rattling around, and you take off the lid and look inside to find hundreds of brightly coloured jigsaw pieces.

Instinctively, you tip the pieces onto your desk and hear them come tumbling out with a clatter as they form a small, haphazard pile. You start to spread the pieces out, noticing how they feel in your hands, whether they're quite thin, flimsy and made of cardboard, or if they're much chunkier and perhaps made of wood. You can feel whether the edges are straight or curved as well as all the bits sticking out waiting to slot neatly into a corresponding piece of the puzzle.

You notice too what the pieces look like, with their different colours, patterns, and shapes; each one showing part of an unknown image that could be one thing or could be something else entirely.

Without a picture on the box to guide you, you think it's going to be very difficult to complete the jigsaw, and there are so many pieces that it feels like a huge challenge in the time you've got available.

But, as you look at the pieces spread out on the desk, you realise that, instead of the picture being hard to imagine, you already know exactly how it should look. And that the pieces will go together however you want them to. You stare more closely now at the multi-coloured mixture of pieces in front of you, and you realise that each one seems bigger than it did at first, and that there are actually far fewer pieces than you initially thought there were.

You realise that, if you stop thinking about the puzzle and just make a start, you can probably finish it quite quickly, and carry on with the rest of your day feeling happy, and with a sense of achievement that a difficult task turned out to be so much easier than you thought it would be. So, you pick up the pieces one by one, running your fingers over the square edges and curved surfaces and you start to slot them easily together.

Beginning in one of the bottom corners, the familiar faces of your family and friends start to take shape and you can clearly see them, smiling and cheering on someone close to them who's with them in the picture.

[*Add some personal details, such as the names of the friends and family who are the biggest support to your client, perhaps with examples of past support offered.*]

In the other bottom corner, as you slot the pieces together, you recognise

[*the place or situation the client wants to change their feelings or behaviour, described as if the change had already taken place.*]

Moving up towards the top of the picture now, you carry on adding the jigsaw pieces more easily and quickly and you see

[*a scene representing the negativity from the past – for example, the school where you were bullied, the labels given to you by your parents, etc.*]

But you know that this is so completely unimportant, and from so long ago, that you barely notice this part of the picture, and you just carry on slotting the other more important pieces into place.

As you reach the final, uppermost corner of the jigsaw, you realise that the few remaining pieces are all different shades of the same colour; a brilliant, vivid yellow. Whether the edges are straight, curved or bumpy, they join together so easily now to complete the puzzle and these final yellow pieces produce such a big and blazing sun high up in the sky that you can actually feel the warmth of its rays and see its beams casting a beautiful, bright light across the whole picture that you've created.

You look closely at the jigsaw once more and see the smiling faces of your supportive family and friends, and the familiar scene, where you are responding in just the way you want to, without being constrained or influenced by feelings and behaviours you had in the past.

And the sun is so dazzling that you can't see anything else in the picture at all. And that doesn't matter. You just feel happy, contented and bathed in sunshine and you know that whatever you do, you can remember this positive feeling and inspiring image and take them with you into your everyday life.

The Author:

Joanne Ainley has a background in local journalism and public relations, which both involve meeting people from all walks of life for all sorts of reasons. These professions depend on being able to communicate with diverse groups and sectors and to grasp exactly what's being described, often without direct experience of the issues involved. Think electric bikes, railway engineering, functional fitness, substance misuse and the impact of spiralling debt – just a snapshot of the unpredictable topics that came her way during previous work.

A natural interest in people and their stories, plus a strong desire to interact with and support individuals to find positive ways forward, led her to a change of direction in 2019. Joanne trained and qualified as a hypnotherapist and has also studied the associated therapy areas of coaching, mindfulness and neuro-linguistic programming (NLP).

RECIPE FOR LIFE

AUTHOR: GEMMA DILLON

Personalisation:

This is a metaphor for those who suffer from perfectionism, especially if it's stress related, and who tend to self-sabotage when things are going well. It refers to a time of change, which could simply be the therapy that they are undertaking, but, of course, you can alter the context to fit your client's situation.

This was written for someone who loved cooking, and that's how it is presented here. Especially if they are a professional, you can refer to them as a chef or baker instead of a cook, or whatever other title seems appropriate.

You could also easily adapt this to refer to other creative pursuits such as art (combining different colours or mediums in a studio), or flower arranging (choosing just the right blooms to go together from a shop, garden or greenhouse).

[Client's name],

you are making changes in your life, and you could not be happier with the decisions you are making. You deserve to enjoy this special time. To cherish it and share it with those you love. But you recognise that, at the moment, things are holding you back from enjoying this time. Things that you still want to change.

I remember you telling me how much you enjoy cooking, so I know that you are a very creative person. You can take separate ingredients and put them together and create beautiful things to make other people happy, whether they are delicious dishes or homemade gifts. You really enjoy that feeling of creating things and bringing pleasure into the lives of those you love. This is one of your special characteristics and talents. So, you are going to use this same talent now to create something to bring pleasure into your own life.

When you are creating your dishes, sometimes you follow a recipe from someone else and sometimes you adapt it to your own tastes. You decide what ingredients you put in, and what you leave out. You add in the ingredients that will enhance the dish, to make it sweeter or richer, and you leave out the ones that would make it too sour, bitter or unpleasant to eat. The good news is that, in exactly the same way as you create these recipes to eat, you can create recipes to live by – 'life recipes' – to live the relaxed, happy and content life you deserve.

Now, I want you to imagine you are standing in your dream kitchen, exactly how you would like it laid out. Perhaps your ideal space is minimal, clean and full of space. Perhaps is it full of all the gadgets and tools you can imagine. It may be quiet, with just you there. Or perhaps you would enjoy being in the bustle of a commercial kitchen where you have commis cooks around to help you, and you can hear these kitchen noises in the background. Take a moment to create your perfect kitchen and enjoy being in there for a while. This is your life kitchen, and it's where you create your life recipes.

Now, I want you to imagine you have a large cooking vessel in front of you, like a large pan. At the moment, this pan is full to the top of nasty, unpleasant ingredients that make you physically tense up and feel uncomfortable. Take a closer look at what is in there:

[*mention examples of thoughts or feelings that are getting in the way of the client's happiness such as perfectionism, agitation, anger, impatience, stress, anxiety, exhaustion, worry, inadequacy, hurt, pain, or sadness.*]

You take a spoon and try to stir it; it is so difficult to stir. Try a bit more. It really is unpleasant. Everything is all clogged up together in the pan, it smells awful, the most disgusting smell you can imagine. This is the recipe you are currently living by. It is not a nice way to live. It is something you want to change. The good news is that you can, and you will ... now ... very easily.

Take a last look at the pan and then I want you to discard it in any way you like. It may be best to put it in the wheelie bin, incinerate it or simply throw it far away into an abyss. Whatever way you wish to dispose of this unpleasant, unhelpful concoction, I would like you to do it now. Give me a little nod when you have done this.

[*Wait for the client's nod.*]

That's great. Feel the relief of getting rid of that awful pan and its contents. You are rid of those nasty, hindering ingredients. They will no longer feature in any of your life recipes.

Now, is the fun part.

I would like you to place yourself firmly in your dream kitchen again and imagine another large cooking vessel in front of you. I'll call it a pan, but you can decide exactly what it looks like to contain your new and improved life recipe.

I'd like you to go around your kitchen and gather all the vital ingredients you know you would like in your new life recipe. Anything that you know will allow you to appreciate your own strengths, have realistic expectations of yourself and others, and allow yourself to enjoy this extra special time in your life. That's it, just go round gathering these ingredients up.

When you are ready you can start adding them to the pan and can go back and get anything you may have forgotten at any time. Maybe you are putting in

[*mention examples of thoughts or feelings that the client has identified as being beneficial, such as patience, excitement, appreciation, calmness, pride, energy, the ability to accept help, and relaxation.*]

Just keep on creating your unique combination. You may like to add a healthy level of self-esteem and self-care as well, topped off with a good dollop of sense of humour!

Whatever you wish to have in there, you can have. Enjoy the process of adding each ingredient. Notice how easily and satisfyingly they blend together. Give it a stir and see how that feels. It feels so good, blending with such ease. Carry on creating your recipe. It feels and smells so good – the most delicious, attractive and fresh smell. Don't forget to put it in the oven for a while, or on the stovetop when you've finished mixing, if it needs that. Do everything you need to, to make it perfect. And when you have finished, give me a nod.

[*Wait for the client's nod.*]

That's brilliant, well done. Notice how it feels to have this positive, fulfilling, energising life recipe in front of you. Notice how it feels throughout your body and take a moment to enjoy the relief and pride of having created this for yourself. You know that this is the recipe you want for your life, and you will keep it going in the future, as easily and enjoyably as you have just experienced.

You now live your life as per this recipe, and it enables you to fulfil your goal of enjoying this special time of change in your life. You understand your value and your worth, and it is not necessary to prove anything to anyone else.

You can deal with setbacks and see them as the bumps they are rather than as 'failures'. And, of course, if you ever feel the need to tweak your recipe, or if you feel that pan needs topping up, then you can easily re-visit your dream kitchen and make any adjustments you need to, for you to continue living free from stress and feelings of inadequacy. You are now free to enjoy living your life for yourself in the way that you want to, embracing happiness and fulfilment.

The Author:

Gemma Dillon has instinctively followed a path to help people. After gaining a Bachelor of Arts (Honours) degree in Counselling Studies in the first ever cohort at York St John's University, she embarked on a career in the National Probation Service. She spent almost eighteen years working for the service to protect the public by directly managing risk, and rehabilitating people in prison and on probation. Gemma moved to a learning and development role, where she delivered training regionally to prison and probation staff on a wide variety of behaviour change and safeguarding programmes. She also designed national training, teaching new staff in the service the fundamentals of developing positive working relationships and evoking positive change for a pro-social future.

Gemma found this to be a rewarding career but, after successfully using hypnotherapy for a variety of issues herself over several years, she became an advocate for its wider use. Gemma came to realise there was no better way to be the ultimate advocate than to train to be a hypnotherapist herself. So, she wasted no time, booked onto the next Yorkshire Hypnotherapy Training practitioner diploma, and trained whilst continuing to work, with three young children and an equally busy husband.

Gemma has been inspired to find that the scope of hypnotherapy benefits is almost boundless and there is always more to learn. Since graduating, Gemma has not looked back and is now making her mark on the hypnotherapy world!

SHOUT OUT
AUTHOR: CLAIRE CASTRO

Personalisation:

T he author says that this fountain story is inspired by an old joke:
three friends are on holiday together, and they come to a big
waterslide where they are told to make a wish on the way down. The first
goes down the slide and says, 'Beer', and lands in a pool of beer. The
second goes down the slide and says, 'Whisky', and lands in a pool of
whisky. The third goes down the slide and says, 'Wheeeeeeeeee!'

In other words, you get what you focus on.

As it's presented here, the focus is on self-esteem and confidence, but
you could change this to pretty much anything your client needed by
adjusting the affirmation.

Use the names of family or friends, if you know them, for the friends
in the story. The protagonist in this story is female, but you can change
the gender to match your client's.

Not for those with a fear of clowns!

[Ask the client, in their mind, to visit their peaceful place, or anywhere
else they feel safe and comfortable before starting.]

While you are sitting there safely and comfortably, I would like to tell you a little story.

Once upon a time, there were three good friends, all

[*give a description of the client, using a broad characteristic, such as 'women in their late twenties'.*]

One day, they met up for a stroll and a day out. They chose to sit on a comfy bench in a warm sunny spot, breathing in the air and saying, 'And relax', and then laughing at their synchronised words.

As they were enjoying a good chat and their picnic, they noticed a nearby fountain, which had a large poster on it. The poster was too small to read from the bench, so they approached it.

The poster said:

Believe it!
1) Repeat the words: 'I love and accept myself' thrice,
2) Shimmy to the left, sashay to the right, shake your hips and fling your arms up, to accept your delight!
3) Make a wish, believe in yourself, and do this right.

And then, there was lots of tiny small-print, which they couldn't read.

Without hesitation, the first woman said confidently, 'I love and accept myself' three times, did the funny dance, and then wished for money. And, lo and behold, she received a caseload of money.

The second woman jumped up next and said confidently, 'I love and accept myself' three times, did the funny dance, and then wished for a holiday to the Caribbean. And, low and behold, she immediately received tickets, with all expenses paid, for a holiday in the Caribbean.

The last friend was not so confident, so she mumbled the words, 'I love and accept myself' three times and did part of the dance half-heartedly. All the while, thinking, 'This is silly, it's embarrassing, it won't work!' Then she couldn't decide what to wish for.

Whilst she was still thinking about it, instead of a wish fulfilled, a clown appeared, with great big, long shoes, baggy trousers, a silly wig, and full clown make-up. He honked a loud horn in the third friend's face and squirted her with water from his silly flower. So silly, so embarrassed.

The other two, seeing their friend's distress, gathered around her, shouting, 'Do it again, change your thoughts and make them good this time! Take three deep breaths, you can do this.'

[*Say the word 'relax' on the client's out breath each time.*]

One, and – relax

Two, and – relax

Three, and – relax.

'Let's shout it out together,' said the first two women, 'Believing it. I love and accept myself, I love and accept myself, I love and accept myself'.

The third friend, helped by the support of the others, began to think happy thoughts, 'I love my friends, I am so lucky to have their support and laughter.'

And, as she thought less about feeling silly and embarrassed, she relaxed, and more happy thoughts appeared, filling her head and whole body with a warm, calm, happy feeling.

The clown disappeared.

'Now, quick, make a better wish!' Her friends shouted, laughing. And she did, she shouted out, did the dance, and got all the confidence she wanted.

And it just goes to show that you can change a negative reaction to your thoughts. You can break the cycle of anxiety. You can acknowledge any uncomfortable thoughts, should they occur, and change them to kinder, more positive ones.

And the more you change your thoughts to positive ones the easier it becomes. You find yourself having more and more positive, happy, kind thoughts. You are retraining your brain to think positive thoughts. It is all within your control, it's your choice.

'Turn your face to the sun, and you do not notice the shadows.'[1]

And if you don't notice the shadows, are they even there?

You have created great coping strategies for life and placed them into your daily routines. Relaxation, exercise, and self-care. You see the positive in every situation, even ones that were once challenging. You know that you have the skills to remain calm, confident, and in control, in any given situation.

[*Ask the client to imagine responding creatively and positively in the future to a specific situation that would have been difficult in the past.*]

You find yourself knowing what you want, and communicating your needs easily. More and more, as time goes on, you adapt to change and have flexible thinking. You look forward to the future with a new zest for life. You are confident, you respect yourself and believe in yourself. You feel a sense of pride, and you feel good about being you. Less reactive. Calm, confident, and in control.

The Author:

Claire has worked as a radiographer for over twenty-eight years in the NHS and the Private sector. She was inspired to train in hypnotherapy after experiencing first-hand how effective it can be for helping with IBS, anxiety and worry.

Thinking hypnotherapy could be applied to help so many others, and wanting to empower people to lead healthier, happier lives, Claire began hypnotherapy training at Yorkshire Hypnotherapy Practitioner Training in 2021 and graduated in July 2022.

She works with a broad range of client issues, including anxiety, stress, relaxation, pain control, hypnobirthing, sports performance, children, weight loss and quitting smoking.

Claire also practises Reiki and runs a holistic service and shop from her home in York and can be found online via www.clairecastrohypnotherapy.com.

Claire believes that everyone loves a story, especially the childlike unconscious mind.

'Stories are a communal currency of humanity,' says Tahir Shar in Arabian Nights.

For centuries, our ancestors have passed on many teachings and much wisdom through metaphors and storytelling. They engage the imagination, creating imagery and igniting emotion in such a gentle, nurturing, indirect way, that the hypnotherapist may broach even the most sensitive of issues.

CHAPTER SEVEN

READINESS FOR CHANGE

According to Prochaska & DiClemente (1983)[1] there are six steps in the cycle of change. These are:

- Precontemplation – essentially before people realise there is a problem, or at least before they know they will have to be proactive to change the situation.
- Contemplation – when people know there is a problem and wonder what to do about it.
- Preparation – the decision-making stage where people start making plans for how to bring about change.
- Action – having decided on a plan, people put the plan into action to create the desired change.
- Maintenance – people work towards keeping the changes in place. Hopefully, this will be a long-term change, but they may move to the next stage.
- Relapse (sometimes) – if people are unable to maintain the changes they've put in place, they will go back to the problem behaviour. This can help provide information about what works (or doesn't) to keep them in the

maintenance stage, as they continue on an upward spiral through the cycle until they successfully achieve long-term maintenance.

DiClemente and Prochaska developed this model whilst working with smokers who wanted to quit, but it has since been applied in many situations, including therapy, social work, drug abuse, bullying, and even encouraging sunscreen or condom use.

It's often said that clients need to be ready for change before it will happen, and if you think they need a bit of a boost to help them get there, these metaphors will help. They're an excellent option for a first session, since they set the scene for the changes that therapy will bring about.

THE FOREST
AUTHOR: BECKY FLEET

Personalisation:

This metaphor works to prepare the client for a natural release of
old behaviours and habits, likening this process to the natural
cycle of trees growing and shedding leaves. Mention a specific forest if you
know of one that the client likes visiting, and include some examples of
habits or thoughts they are ready to shed.

So, as you gently relax there now, I want you to imagine you're at
the edge of a beautiful forest.

It's a warm comfortable day, the sky is an amazing shade of
blue, and the cheerful sun smiles down on you. The warm rays are
so comforting as they caress your face, and you become aware of a
soft breeze. The breeze teases you with the scents from the forest,
and the sound of the leaves whispers a welcome to you and invites
you to explore the beauty of the woods.

You begin to walk lazily along the forest path; it's easy
underfoot, and the soft mosses release their fresh earthy aroma. As
you walk deeper into the woods, you find yourself experiencing the
forest with all your senses, you become aware of the sounds of the

forest, the gentle snapping of twigs under your feet, the soft whispering of the leaves, the friendly birdsong celebrating the beauty of the day.

You continue to walk slowly, going deeper and deeper, slowing down, taking a few moments to inhale the fresh clean air and the scent of the trees, letting it nourish and revive you.

[*Pause.*]

It's so satisfying to watch how the sunlight dances and plays through the canopy of the trees. The ever-changing contrast of light and shade provides a kaleidoscope of shapes and colours, a whole spectrum of healing green light.

You come to a small clearing and notice an old fallen tree trunk. The sun's rays have warmed its surface and the bark is smooth and worn beneath your hands, it's the perfect place to sit and rest for a while.

You feel totally content here, so peaceful and calm, knowing there's nobody here but you. Nobody asking anything from you, nobody expecting anything, no decisions to make, this is just the perfect place for you to relax.

You settle down here to enjoy the moment, taking comfort in peacefully observing the forest life, as it quietly continues around you, the sounds of the birds in the trees, the rustling and scampering of rabbits and squirrels, and butterflies dancing through shafts of light.

The soft scents of the fresh forest air waft over you, an intoxicating and delicious blend of flowers, trees, and earth. All the life of the forest, existing and living together, symbiotic in their harmony.

And relaxing here in complete tranquillity, you can feel the power of nature, the life energy flowing all around you. It's everywhere, yet silent and unseen. You're aware of the essence of life that floods the forest, continually flowing beneath your feet to be carried from deep within the soil, through the roots of the trees, to the smallest leaf on the highest treetop.

The forest, and all the life within it, uses its energy effectively and efficiently, controlling and focusing its use and its outputs, so easily and naturally that growth, strength, and resilience are unavoidable.

Look around you at the forest and feel how the energy is shared out effectively between all the living things. The shade-loving plants grow steadily within the shelter of the trees, whilst those that need sunlight grow tall and climb towards the sun.

The forest instinctively knows where to focus its energy. In the depths of winter, it cuts back its leaves, conserving its energy while there is less light. But, even during these times, the energy is still flowing, directed and focused on new growth, ready to utilise the power of the sun, when it returns.

The energy is hidden secretly within closed buds as they embrace the growth within, preparing to showcase their beauty.

Those new, fresh, vibrant leaves might grow slowly at first, just a small shoot, then a bud, and as they develop, they unfurl into the most wonderful shapes and colours, filling the forest canopy and flourishing until the seasons change.

And, as autumn arrives, the continual cycle of growth and replenishment continues, and with each cycle, the trees become stronger and more resilient. Those leaves that were so fresh at one point are no longer necessary for the tree; it's time for the next cycle to begin.

The trees drop their leaves when they are no longer of use. There is no resistance or doubt, the trees have a job to do, and they naturally perform that task. They release those leaves to fall gently and easily to the ground. When the tree decides it's time to let go, it doesn't hold onto those leaves; they are released and are now a part of its past.

And, in nature, there is no waste, the past is never wasted, only transformed.

The old leaves gather on the forest floor, releasing any remaining nutrients into the soil, to nurture and be recycled into the new growth.

Relaxing so deeply there, it's almost as if you've become

blended with the forest, at one with nature. The energy flows from beneath you, and through you, rejuvenating and restoring you, rebalancing your thoughts, providing clarity, and calming your mind. Like the trees, you can release the past and look forward to new growth, new ideas, and new feelings. Nothing wasted, no learning released, simply words, thoughts, and feelings whose time has passed.

[*Mention some personal examples.*]

It's so comforting to be here, feeling completely relaxed, knowing these things will happen. Ready for them to happen. Excited to see that change taking place, naturally and easily.

It's so refreshing to experience such total peace within yourself, and you take note of how good this feels, saving the memory so you can revisit this feeling within your mind whenever you need to.

And when you come back to your daily life ... at the end of this session, you'll feel so much calmer and more balanced than you have for a long time. And every time you take a deep breath and think about this forest experience you find clarity and focus in your thoughts.

The Author:

Becky Fleet of New Approach Hypnotherapy is based in Huddersfield in West Yorkshire, and also offers online sessions.

Becky has spent over twenty-five years working in corporate environments, during which she supported many colleagues through stress, anxiety, and burnout. Hypnotherapy was something that Becky always had a keen interest in. So, when pregnant with her first child, it was almost inevitable that she turned to Hypnobirthing for support. Through this experience, Becky saw that hypnotherapy could also be used to help others through a wide range of life scenarios and fulfilled a need that was especially unmet within the corporate world.

Becky was keen to offer this help and chose to study hypnotherapy with Yorkshire Hypnotherapy Training. The diverse course content, the high quality of teaching, and the requirement to deliver hours of face-to-face therapy before qualifying as a hypnotherapist all ensured that Becky was able to provide help to clients presenting with a wide range of issues, from the outset.

Becky is very much a 'people person' and enjoys working with all clients, adapting sessions to provide individually focused solutions. Although clients might present with similar issues, everybody has a different story to tell, and it's only by working together that the best ending can be achieved.

Becky feels there is nothing more satisfying for both the client and the therapist than experiencing the very real changes that hypnotherapy can accomplish.

THE RADIO

AUTHOR: HILARY RICHARDSON

Personalisation:

R adios are fun to play around with as metaphors. The words coming from them represent the internal dialogue the client is experiencing, and the channel (or the announcer) can be changed, they can be switched to a new channel or turned off altogether.

You can, of course, alter the environment in which the client is listening, for example, making it a car radio if the client is experiencing driving anxiety, or an MP3 player or iPod if you think that will resonate more. Swap out words like 'hope and positivity' for words your client uses to describe what they want to experience.

You can also make the protagonist female if your client identifies that way or give them a name that sounds a bit like the client's, to help them recognise themselves in the story.

I am going to share with you a story about a man and his radio. This man was a keen radio listener. Ever since he could remember, he had sat and listened to the same radio programme. It was the channel of his youth and the wavelength of his life.

He always sat in the same chair to listen. There was a comfort in sitting in his own familiar chair, surrounded by the objects and furnishings he had always known. Everything in its usual place, nothing new, nothing different, everything unchanged.

Every day he ensured he was tuned in to the same channel and listened to the dark stories, the depressing debates, and the melancholy music.

[*Insert an example of programmes based on the client's negative internal dialogue.*]

The radio announcer's voice was dull and flat. The man often felt utter despair, but it was what he always listened to. It had become a way of life.

Often the heavy feeling of misery weighed him down. This was his wavelength though, his channel, his programme. He had been brought up listening to this channel, so listen he did. He took in every word and every note of the miserable music. The debates left him feeling worried and nervous. He carried the worry, the nerves, and the feeling of despair everywhere with him. The world was a difficult place. He knew this for sure because of the wavelength he was tuned into.

One day, he switched on the radio and found it was tuned in to a different channel. It was a big surprise, but the upbeat voice of the announcer caused him to stay with it for a while. He listened to jolly music, amusing and inspiring discussions, and stories that made him feel good.

[*Insert a positive example based on what the client wants their internal dialogue to sound like.*]

In fact, he began to laugh out loud at some of the stories and, as he laughed, he felt a feeling of release. A weight being lifted. Some fantastic things were going on in the world. He listened to upbeat articles and felt new feelings of hope and positivity. He was on a new frequency.

He realised that this new channel could be his new wavelength. He had a new programme. The old programme was not pre-set, and as he sat in his own familiar chair, he looked out at the objects and furnishings around him. Everything was in its usual place, but there was something new and there was something different. There was change.

The man felt a sense of vibrancy within, a sense of control. He could easily control the wavelength of his life, and benefit from the change of channel. New channels could be explored. He became excited about the change.

Change is inevitable. The old channels are there but we can always explore new programmes, change wavelengths, and tune into new and more beneficial messages. Have a new and better soundtrack to your life. You are worth it. You deserve to be the best version of yourself. You are in control of what you choose to listen to.

Soon, I will bring you back to full consciousness and you will feel empowered, liberated, strong and ready right now for positive change.

The Author:

Hilary Richardson is a hypnotherapist with a special passion for working with children. She lives with her husband and a small menagerie in Horsforth, Leeds and is the owner of Introspicere Hypnotherapy. Hilary has worked at a senior level in childcare for over thirty years where she spreads her passion for play. Her motto is that all children who are, and have been, in her care will remember her with happiness. Hilary is a serial course-goer and has gained many certifications and qualifications in her pursuit to offer Best Practices.

When she is not working, Hilary enjoys writing, dog walking, collecting items for her house – which is 1950s authentically furnished and decorated – and meditating. Hilary is a proud mum to grown-up twins and grandma to three lively boys.

Her favourite quote is that 'The glass is neither half full, nor is it half empty – it is just refillable', which is another metaphor you can use with your clients!

THE SHRINKING ISLAND

AUTHOR: RACHEL GOTH

Personalisation:

his is a metaphor for change and developing the courage to make it come about, but it also talks about following your own path and not becoming too dependent on other people's approval. It's a good metaphor where you think resistance might be playing a part in sustaining the client's issues, or where there is secondary gain (a benefit, often unconscious, in continuing the problem).

As with many of these stories, you can change the gender of the protagonist to match the client, and replace words like 'hope and excitement' with words the client uses about their own feelings as they reach their goal.

Far, far away, in the middle of the sea stood an island. The island was populated by a community of people who had lived there for too many generations to remember. Their history was passed on from father to son, mother to daughter, in stories and songs told by the elders.

They spoke of how their people had originally travelled to the island, fleeing a terrible monster who had tyrannised them on the mainland and kept them living in fear. Moving to the island had been the beginning of a new chapter for the community. The island was their saviour, a nirvana that the monster could not follow due to its fear of the sea.

The island had provided for the people's every need and the people worshipped it in return, with festivals and days of thanks. An abundance of nutritious fruits and vegetables sustained them. Fresh springs provided water, and beautiful forests were their shelter. The community wanted for nothing. They soon came to think of themselves as islanders and, as the generations went by, the land of their origin faded from memory.

But the only constant in life is change and, slowly but surely, over the millennia, the sea began to nibble away at the island's edge as it ebbed and flowed, flowed and ebbed. Eroding a cliff here, a shoreline there. Taking chunks of forest, tumbling down into the sea. And, over the years, many of their homes were lost to the waves.

The people adapted as much as they could, building defences along the coastline where the waves were harshest, and designing homes on stilts to withstand the rising water. But eventually, they were forced to move deeper into the island, away from their beloved lush forests and fresh-water springs. And each year there was less land to forage and farm, fewer trees for shelter, and more springs and wells lost to the sea. And moving home each season became a way of life.

One day, a young woman of the community was collecting her possessions to move once again when, not for the first time, her attention was taken by the land across the sea. That land was wide and vast, with an abundance of forest. The woman wondered if it had fresh water, and food too. If it had all those things, then maybe it could be a new home for her people.

She'd put the idea to the elders before, but they had refused to even consider it. There was a reason their ancestors had moved to the island, they said. There were monsters on the mainland, just waiting for new prey. And it wasn't going to be them!

Perhaps the monsters were long gone, she'd suggested, but the elders were having none of it. 'Have you not heard the horrendous sounds that drift across the ocean from that place?' they said.

The woman suggested they send over a search party in a small boat to investigate. They could check for monsters and let the rest of the islanders know if it would make a good new home. After all, their island wouldn't be habitable for much longer.

'No,' the elders said; their ancestors had moved to this island for a reason and that is where they would stay.

Then, one day, distraught by the plight of her people, and frustrated by the stubbornness of the elders, the woman decided to take matters into her own hands. Secretly, she began to collect supplies to journey to the mainland until, one night, she'd gathered enough and decided it was time to leave. So, she waited until the rest of the community were asleep before creeping down to the water's edge, where she set sail in a tiny fishing boat.

With only the light of the moon to guide her, at times she found herself in complete darkness, waiting for the clouds to pass. But she held to her goal. One way or another, she would know if this could be a new home for her people. And, comforted by the possibility of finding an abundance of fruits, vegetables, shelter, and water, she held thoughts of the monsters at bay and kept on sailing towards the distant land.

At times, the wind dropped, the sails flagged, and she thought about turning back. But, instead, she took out her oars and rowed on. At other times, the boat glided so swiftly towards its destination on the currents, a great fear rose inside her at the thought of what she might find. But she turned her thoughts towards all the good things she might find, and the future she could have with her people.

There were points when she felt full of hope and excitement, and times when she wondered if she was making a mistake, yet she moved forward bit by bit.

Eventually, after what felt like days, the sun began to rise, and the boat arrived in the shallows of the mysterious land. She waded onto the shore and made her way towards the forest, where the first thing she noticed was the sounds which so scared the elders of her village. But they didn't seem so ferocious from close up, and she was curious as to what they could be.

As she entered the forest, the sounds became louder and louder, and she began to wonder if the elders were right. But she steeled herself to continue. For a while, she couldn't see where the din was coming from and then, suddenly, out of the trees swished a dozen birds, their colourful feathers gleaming in the sunlight. They were very noisy indeed, but equally beautiful as they glided across the forest canopy.

Next, she spied some familiar fruits, mangoes with ripe and juicy flesh, their fragrance filling her nostrils. And, after a few more hours of exploring, she'd found plenty of fresh spring water to quench her thirst, foods to forage, and places suitable for planting and shelter. She took some of the fruits and water with her and hurried back to her boat, eager to tell the rest of the community what she'd found.

Many of the islanders were overjoyed to see her return, especially with her good news about the mainland. But not all the islanders were pleased to see her. The elders called her a liar, and some even said she was in league with the monsters, trying to lure them to their destruction. So, when she set sail again for the land of plenty, not everyone accompanied her, but she took comfort in the fact she was helping those she could.

A few months later, as the island shrank smaller and smaller, a new colony was firmly established on the mainland. And the people there grew healthier, happier, and stronger than ever, having found everything they needed.

And the woman concentrated her attention on the new colony, doing her best to help it flourish. She hoped that one day the rest would join them in their new nirvana, but she knew that that would have to be their decision. She was content, accepting that she could only help those who were willing to be helped.

The Author:

Rachel Goth is a trained master coach and hypnotherapist, who specialises in helping coaches, therapists and teachers learn to love their voice, so they can share their message without having to change the way they speak.

She knows first-hand what it's like learning to use your voice for your business, show up as yourself on social media and create recordings for your clients. She now helps her clients to do the same by helping them move from disliking their voices to becoming confident in the way they sound.

Through a combination of 1:1 coaching, and practical exercises, Rachel helps her clients establish a new positive belief in their voice, so they feel confident being themselves and sharing their message. Within a couple of weeks, her clients are confidently recording their own meditations, creating courses, and ad-libbing their social media videos with ease.

Find out more at rachelgoth.com

CHAPTER EIGHT

MINI METAPHORS

Finally, I was inspired to include a few mini metaphors by this one from Raymond Bergner.[1]

#1: A lion walks in the room ... Pat feels scared ... Pat takes a happy pill ... Pat doesn't feel scared anymore ... the lion eats Pat.

#2: A lion walks in the room ... Mike freezes in panic ... Mike takes a happy pill ... Mike unfreezes ... Mike runs out the back door and escapes the lion.

It's a bit tongue in cheek, however, the point is made. Sometimes therapy (like 'happy pills') is not enough on its own to resolve a situation, but it does help you do what you need to do.

All the metaphors in this chapter are less than 300 words.

This is a mini chapter as well, but I hope it's enough to give you some ideas for a few mini metaphors of your own. And if you haven't yet read the Telling Stories article at the beginning of this book, go and look through it now. The cup of tea story works very well as a mini metaphor, and you're welcome to borrow it.

Mini metaphors can often be inspired by everyday experiences with your family, car, or pets – perhaps they are the Country and Western song side of metaphor creation?

Or take note of words or phrases that your client uses. Look for comments like, 'My heart is heavy', 'I can't see a way forward' or 'Nothing makes sense'. (That last one brings *Alice in Wonderland* into my mind – what about you? Or *The Matrix*, perhaps?)

Brainstorm what that phrase could mean if it was literally true and go from there.

AEROPLANES
AUTHOR: DEBBIE WALLER

Personalisation:

T his is about letting go and allowing the negative influences of the past to fade. It could be brought into the client's peaceful place or used as a standalone.

You could also, depending on the client's interests, use footprints in sand, snow, or mud, or perhaps the wake of a boat, to make the point that the past can be seen, for a while, but, in the future, we can choose to diverge from that path.

Have you ever looked up into the sky on a summer's day and seen a white, gauzy trail left by an aeroplane?

They're called contrails, and although they look like smoke, they're really made of ice crystals, formed by the warm exhaust from the plane hitting the cooler air around it.

Sometimes you see the contrail and you can't see the plane at all, because contrails can last a while, clearly marking where the plane has travelled, even when it's moved on.

It's like being able to see into the past, the whole journey that the plane has made.

But the nice thing is that the plane can go anywhere it likes, seeing the past behind it, but free to change direction until the contrail fades and all you can see is the blue of the open sky.

The Author:

Debbie Waller is a hypnotherapist in Normanton, West Yorkshire. She is also a hypnotherapy supervisor and Director/Head Tutor of Yorkshire Hypnotherapy Training. She is the author of 'Their Worlds, Your Words', and 'The Hypnotherapist's Companion', a contributor to the 'Hypnotherapy Handbook' and past editor of the 'Hypnotherapy Journal'. And of course, contributing editor of this book of metaphors.

AURA

AUTHOR: HILARY RICHARDSON

Personalisation:

An adaptation of the 'protective bubble' theme, this could have gone into the 'Twists on the Classics' chapter but, by virtue of its brevity, it is here instead.

Because of the word aura, this is most suited to clients who have an interest in spirituality, holistic health, and similar areas, and/or you can combine it with a nature-based peaceful place. Make the light their favourite colour if you know what that is.

You can finish by anchoring the good feelings if you wish, so the client has access to them at any time.

Witness yourself enjoying the fresh and fragrant scents of the woods; the perfume of the flowers; the uplifting smell of foliage – green and strong, growing.

Nature helps to ensure the plants and trees grow strong and sturdy. Here, in nature, you feel free, you feel strong, and you feel optimistic, and, as you find yourself at one with nature, take a moment to enjoy the experience of your mind and body feeling so strong, feeling so comfortable, and so relaxed.

I want to ask you to sense a vibrant light, shining positively, and surrounding your body.

Feel that positive energy. Be aware of how calm you feel. Do you notice yet how it surrounds your whole body?

This is your special protective aura. It maintains your positive energy. It is always there for you.

Its brightness can deflect any unwanted thoughts and feelings. Anytime you have thoughts that are less than good, you imagine this aura emanating from you and protecting you from those negative thoughts and feelings.

The more you believe in your protective aura, the stronger it will become. It brings health and happiness to your mind, and to your body. You can choose to feel protected by your aura anytime you need to.

And, because you feel so free from negative thoughts by simply imagining your aura, you choose to feel positive, resilient, and calm at all times.

The Author:

Hilary Richardson is a hypnotherapist with a special passion for working with children. She lives with her husband and a small menagerie in Horsforth, Leeds and is the owner of Introspicere Hypnotherapy. Hilary has worked at a senior level in childcare for over thirty years where she spreads her passion for play. Her motto is that all children who are, and have been, in her care will remember her with happiness. Hilary is a serial course-goer and has gained many certifications and qualifications in her pursuit to offer Best Practices.

When she is not working, Hilary enjoys writing, dog walking, collecting items for her house – which is 1950s authentically furnished and decorated – and meditating. Hilary is a proud mum to grown-up twins and grandma to three lively boys.

Her favourite quote is that 'The glass is neither half full, nor is it half empty – it is just refillable', which is another metaphor you can use with your clients!

BORIS AND THE WHEEL

AUTHOR: DEBBIE WALLER

Personalisation:

B est for clients who like animals and especially those who are not freaked out by mice and rats, for whom a hamster might be just too close! Having said that, if they have a pet of their own of the sort that might run on a wheel, you could easily change Boris's species to whatever you felt was most appropriate!

This is a good metaphor for people who talk about being trapped in pointless routines, 'running on the spot' or 'never getting anywhere' since that's exactly what happens on a hamster wheel. You could personalise it by adding in some examples of what their own 'wheel' might be; the tasks they never seem to complete. You could also use a similar story about a person exercising on a treadmill if your client liked going to the gym. Running forever but travelling nowhere.

As it stands, this story is based on truth (we've had lots of pets over the years), but feel free to use it as it is, even if you never had a hamster. Presenting it as a memory sets some context, though, plus it's Boris's one chance for immortality!

. . .

When I was a child, we had a Russian hamster, a little grey and silver one named Boris. He liked to play on his hamster wheel, running faster and faster. Sometimes he would go so fast that, when he stopped running, it continued to spin, strongly enough to flip him out of the wheel or to send him upside down, right over the top.

In the wild, hamsters run up to five miles a night to find food, but no matter how much effort Boris put into running on his wheel, he never got anywhere. It was good exercise and he seemed to enjoy it, at least for a while, but, in the end, he just went round in circles.

Some hamsters get addicted to their wheels, so they continue to run even after their feet are sore, but Boris knew better. Fear of the consequences, like being flipped off or tipped upside down, never prevented him from stopping the wheel when he'd had enough. He would go for a nap, trundle through his tunnels, climb up ladders, and forage for the food and treats we'd hidden around his home to make life more interesting.

He knew it was okay to stop running in circles and getting nowhere. It was okay to do something more productive, or even to take a rest. And you can do that too. You can make new choices instead of constantly wasting your energy in a way that doesn't take you forward.

[*Include some personal examples from what the client has told you.*]

Give yourself permission, right now, to get off the wheel, prioritise what matters to you, and do the things that take you towards your goals.

The Author:

Debbie Waller is a hypnotherapist in Normanton, West Yorkshire. She is also a hypnotherapy supervisor and Director/Head Tutor of Yorkshire Hypnotherapy Training. She is the author of 'Their Worlds, Your Words', and 'The Hypnotherapist's Companion', a contributor to the 'Hypnotherapy Handbook' and past editor of the 'Hypnotherapy Journal'. And of course, contributing editor of this book of metaphors.

TEFLON AND VELCRO
AUTHOR: LARA MCCLURE

Personalisation:

A n initial brainstorm is required to establish what proven skills and acknowledged personal qualities are already in place to help the client to tackle their presenting issue, and to identify who in their life might support and encourage them (this is of course a therapeutic process in itself!)

If the client struggles to identify any suitable personal resources, you can work with them on developing these strengths before using this metaphor.

These can then all be emphasised as sticking to the mind like Velcro, while the negative self-talk that is preventing the client from tackling the issue successfully is sent sliding off the mind like Teflon.

Any worries you might have about
[*presenting issue*]
will simply slide out of your mind as if it were made of Teflon; they simply cannot stick there. All the positive things that you know about your ability to do
[*presenting issue*]

using

[*existing skills*]

skills and

[*existing personal qualities*]

– these stick in your mind as if they were made of Velcro.

All the praise, support and encouragement you receive from others,

[*give specific examples*]

this, too, sticks in your Velcro mind.

And you will find that you are easily able to use both qualities of your mind, the Teflon mind that allows unhelpful thoughts to easily slip away, and the Velcro mind that instinctively clings on to useful ideas that reinforce your personal power.

You are capable, you are strong, and you know what you want to do. You have the skill and ability you need to achieve this, and you have the support around you. The certainty of this holds firm in your Velcro mind and you find yourself easily and effortlessly achieving your goals.

The Author:

Lara McClure came to hypnotherapy through storytelling, and her practice is strongly rooted in that craft, finding profound therapeutic potential in carefully constructed bespoke narratives. Lara enjoys creating unique thoughtscapes to help individuals make positive changes in their lives. She loves a good metaphor as a creative and non-confrontational way to approach an issue sideways, which the subconscious mind instinctively 'gets'!

Lara is passionate about the evidence basis for her work and will often direct clients to scientific papers supporting the techniques used in their therapy. She teaches research methodology to students of acupuncture and Chinese Herbal Medicine at the Northern College of Acupuncture in York, and loves how judicious use of evidence can support therapeutic decision-making, and enhance the credibility of Complementary Therapies, an irresistible balance of science and art.

Lara is a mum to three and a Nana to two (so far!). She currently practises hypnotherapy in Pocklington, North Yorkshire in a multidisciplinary practice alongside acupuncturists and bodyworkers

- https://www.learntoheal.uk/team/lara-mcclure.

RESOURCES

If you have enjoyed this book, please leave a review on Amazon.

And check out these other resources from Debbie Waller

Books

The Hypnotherapist's Companion: a practical guide to practice
Their Worlds, Your Words: the hypnotherapist's guide to effective scripts and sessions
The Hypnotherapy Handbook, ed: Ann Jaloba (contributor)
All available from Amazon in paperback and on kindle
Or you can buy direct from the author via www.debbiewaller-author.co.uk

Online

Hypnotherapy Training & Practitioner Magazine
https://hypnotherapytrainingblog.blogspot.com/
Free articles by Debbie Waller on business building, client work, and more.

Contact Debbie Waller

Please feel free to contact Debbie Waller about training, supervision or CPD.

https://debbiewallerauthor.co.uk

https://yorkshirehypnotherapytraining.co.uk

https://cpd.expert

INDEX BY AUTHOR

INDEX BY TITLE

Readers please note: 'the' is ignored for alphabetising

NOTES

Stories, meaning and metaphor

1. Cited in Parkinson, R (2001) The Healing History of Therapeutic Storytelling. [Blog] Mark Tyrrell's Therapy Skills. Available at: https://www.unk.com/blog/the-healing-history-of-therapeutic-storytelling/.
2. Wikipedia Contributors (2019). Sun. [online] Wikipedia. Available at: https://en.wikipedia.org/wiki/Sun.
3. Matthews, A. (2017). Mother demands son's school ban Sleeping Beauty. [online] Mail Online. Available at: https://www.dailymail.co.uk/news/article-5110415/Mother-demands-son-s-school-ban-Sleeping-Beauty.html [Accessed 10 Jun. 2022].
4. Grady, C. (2018). Kristen Bell has some doubts about Snow White and consent. She's part of a long tradition. [online] Vox. Available at: https://www.vox.com/culture/2018/10/19/17995442/snow-white-history-evolution-consent-kristen-bell [Accessed 10 Jun. 2022].
5. www.imdb.com. (n.d.). Jurassic Park (1993) – IMDb. [online] Available at: https://www.imdb.com/title/tt0107290/characters/nm0000368 [Accessed 10 Jun. 2022].
6. SparkNotes. (n.d.). Animal Farm: Questions & Answers. [online] Available at: https://www.sparknotes.com/lit/animalfarm/key-questions-and-answers/.
7. Kambury, R. (2017). War Without Allegory: WWI, Tolkien, and The Lord of the Rings – World War I Centennial. [online] Worldwar1centennial.org. Available at: https://www.worldwar1centennial.org/index.php/articles-posts/5502-war-not-allegory-wwi-tolkien-and-the-lord-of-the-rings.html.

Stories and the brain

1. The Storyteller Agency. (n.d.). 50 Best Quotes for Storytelling. [online] Available at: https://thestorytelleragency.com/goodreads/50-best-quotes-for-storytelling.
2. Zak PJ. Why inspiring stories make us react: the neuroscience of narrative. Cerebrum. 2015 Feb 2;2015:2. PMID: 26034526; PMCID: PMC4445577.
3. Brockington, G., Moreira, A.P.G., Buso, M.S., Silva, S.G. da, Altszyler, E., Fischer, R. and Moll, J. (2021). Storytelling increases oxytocin and positive emotions and decreases cortisol and pain in hospitalized children. Proceedings of the National Academy of Sciences, [online] 118(22). doi:10.1073/pnas.2018409118.

4. Lai, Vicky T. Howerton, Olivia. Desai, Rutvik H. Concrete processing of action metaphors: Evidence from ERP. Brain Research, 2019; 1714: 202 DOI: 10.1016/j.brainres.2019.03.005

Using therapeutic stories and metaphors

1. www.goodreads.com. (n.d.). A quote by Ben Okri. [online] Available at: https://www.goodreads.com/quotes/7421473-beware-of-the-stories-you-read-or-tell-subtly-at [Accessed 10 Jun. 2022].
2. ResearchGate. (n.d.). (PDF) Therapeutic Storytelling Revisited. [online] Available at: https://www.researchgate.net/publication/6080623_Therapeutic_Storytelling_Revisited.
3. De La Torre, J. (1972). The therapist tells a story: A technique in brief psychotherapy. Bulletin of the Menninger Clinic, 36, 606-616

Become a better storyteller

1. Bergner, Raymond. (2007). Therapeutic Storytelling Revisited. (Page 4) American journal of psychotherapy. 61. 149-62. 10.1176/appi. psychotherapy.2007.61.2.149.

Making metaphors of your own

1. The Storyteller Agency. (n.d.). 50 Best Quotes for Storytelling. [online] Available at: https://thestorytelleragency.com/goodreads/50-best-quotes-for-storytelling.
2. in Flanagan, John Sommers (2019). Using Therapeutic Storytelling with Children: Five Easy Steps. [online] John Sommers-Flanagan. Available at: https://johnsommersflanagan.com/2019/07/08/using-therapeutic-storytelling-with-children-five-easy-steps/.

Chapter Two

1. Source: Goodreads.com. (2020). A quote from Mark Twain's Own Autobiography. [online] Available at: https://www.goodreads.com/quotes/843880-there-is-no-such-thing-as-a-new-idea-it.

Cinderella

1. Cox, Marian Roalfe (1893). Cinderella: Three Hundred and Forty-five Variants of Cinderella, Catskin, and Cap O' Rushes. London: The Folklore Society.

Elysian Fields

1. The Rainbow Bridge is a wonderful place full of trees, flowers and meadows just this side of Heaven where pets of all kinds who have passed out of this life wait for their owners, so they can cross into Heaven together. Find out more on their website: https://www.rainbowsbridge.com
2. A metaphor for life and death, preparing the client for what is to come.
3. Tholos is an ancient circular temple; again, it might not be a good word for you to use if your client isn't likely to be familiar with it. You could easily substitute it for a gazebo or a structure of your choice.

Shout Out

1. This phrase has been credited to many sources, from being 'an old Māori saying', to a quote from Walt Whitman or Helen Keller. The exact origin is unclear, according to Quote Investigator, (2019). Keep Your Face Always Towards the Sunshine, and the Shadows Will Fall Behind You – Quote Investigator. [online] Available at: https://quoteinvestigator.com/2019/03/05/sunshine/ [Accessed 3 Jun. 2022].

Chapter Seven

1. Yeshiva. (2021). Prochaska and DiClemente's Stages of Change Model for Social Workers. [online] Available at: https://online.yu.edu/wurzweiler/blog/prochaska-and-diclementes-stages-of-change-model-for-social-workers-2.

Chapter Eight

1. Bergner, Raymond. (2007). Therapeutic Storytelling Revisited. American journal of psychotherapy. 61. 149-62. 10.1176/appi.psychotherapy.2007.61.2.149. ('Two lions' story on P 12, said to be adapted from Ossorio, 1997).

Ingram Content Group UK Ltd.
Milton Keynes UK
UKHW011943170723
425287UK00008B/445